Last Served?

Social Aspects of AIDS

Series Editor: Peter Aggleton
Goldsmiths' College, University of London

Last Served?
Gendering the HIV Pandemic

Cindy Patton

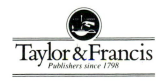

Taylor & Francis
Publishers since 1798

UK	Taylor & Francis Ltd, 4 John St., London WC1N 2ET
USA	Taylor & Francis Inc., 1900 Frost Road, Suite 101, Bristol, PA 19007

First published 1994

A Catalogue Record for this book is available from the British Library

ISBN 0 7484 0189 X
ISBN 0 7484 0190 3 (pbk)

Library of Congress Cataloging-in-Publication Data are available on request

Series Cover design by Barking Dog Art, additional artwork by Hybert • Design & Type.

Typeset in 12/13pt Baskerville
by Franklin Graphics, Lord Street, Southport

Printed in Great Britain by Burgess Science Press, Basingstoke on paper which has a specified pH value on final paper manufacture of not less than 7.5 and is therefore 'acid free'.

Contents

Series Editor's Preface

Contrary to the impression given by some early prevention efforts, AIDS is not an 'equal opportunities' disease, affecting everyone and all communities equally. Indeed, one of the most striking characteristics of the epidemic has been its capacity to reinforce existing social inequalities — of gender, of social status, of race, and of sexuality.

Last Served? examines these concerns in detail, focusing particularly on women's positioning in the epidemic — discursively as the subjects of epidemiology; economically in the international and domestic spheres; and politically as individuals and communities affected by patriarchy. It highlights the nature and complexity of women's vulnerability to infection, as well as the burden they carry as care givers and as educators.

Drawing on more than a decade's experience in AIDS activism and organising, and utilising the techniques offered by contemporary cultural analysis and theory, Cindy Patton offers a dramatically new appreciation of the ways in which women are responding to the challenge of AIDS in the developing as well as the developed world.

Peter Aggleton

Introduction

It is now clear that there is significant international concern about women in the HIV/AIDS pandemic. Recent national and international AIDS conferences have had unprecedented numbers of presentations about women and AIDS, and there are many formal and informal projects for and sometimes by women at risk of contracting HIV. Once considered an issue marginal to the 'real' thrust of the epidemic, raising the question of women at risk of contracting HIV is no longer controversial. But it is still not easy: getting women's needs addressed is still not automatic because conflicting constructions of gender form the basis of the very logic through which science, the media, educators and policymakers operate.

A generous reconstruction of the response to women's needs in the epidemic would suggest that there was confusion, mislabeling, and understandable, if misguided, effort to prioritize programming to the clearest areas of caseload. But this account would be profoundly untrue: 'women' were not overlooked in the frenzy of a public health emergency. News writers and researchers relied on longstanding cultural constructions of women which take a minimal (but, obviously, highly problematic) notion of the 'sexed' body — the (female) reproductive body — and add connotative meanings associated with sexual appropriateness — heterosexual and monogamous. AIDS discourse extended to the world this prudish, racist, and class-linked US construction of 'woman' which had for two centuries served to protect sex-role-conforming women of the white middle class, while heaping abuse on all other women. Thus, instead of accepting the often circulated idea that women were 'invisible' in the first decade of the epidemic, I want to argue that particular and specific ways of carving up the category 'woman' into a series of women-who-do-not-count-as-women was fundamental to the original paradigm through which researchers, policymakers, educators, and the media first understood the AIDS epidemic.

While the increasing number of books and articles on 'women and AIDS' and the general trend toward more openly acknowledging and planning for women are causes for optimism, there is still much to be done. The greater visibility of 'women' cannot quickly or easily change the underlying assumptions which simultaneously made woman both a radiant figure of sexual purity and a magnet for blame during the pandemic's first decade. The fundamental divides posed in the current ideology of 'limited resources' pits women against men or each other: gay men versus women of color; drug-injecting males versus women who inject or who have sex with them; women in the unplanned dimensions of developing economies versus women in domestic spheres. These complex, gendered oppositions inhibit women's attempts to work together; impede the creation of meaningful alliances with the men whose experience of the epidemic is also inscribed through gendered constructions; and prevent empowering collaboration between women and the policymakers and educators operating within the current epidemiological categories.

Women's position in the epidemic is understood radically differently depending on whether women's concerns are posed by governments of developed or developing countries, by gay-community-dominated or racial/ethnic-community-dominated groups, by women influenced by the women's health movement or by women influenced principally by AIDS activism. One of the purposes of this book is to make clearer how the differing ways of posing and answering questions about women and HIV are grounded in existing ways of thinking about gender issues. These differences relate to political and economic structures, as well as to the possibilities women have seized for resisting the forms of domination which undeniably surround them. I doubt that these differences in understanding women's status can be fully reconciled to produce anything like a single political project or global strategy. Nevertheless, I hope my suggestions about some of the sources of difference will be useful in understanding the requirements for any alliance.

Thinking Gender

In this book I hope to make a particular kind of contribution to the growing literature on women and AIDS. Other books have gathered together current knowledge about women's situation in the HIV pandemic, an extremely important advance, but different than the focus of this volume. Instead of enumerating the *effects* on women of confused or conflicting constructions of gender — effects which are devastating and immoral, and which it is vital to reverse — this book describes how *particular* ideas about gender emerged and have informed representations of and policy for women in the HIV epidemic. Instead of replacing invisibility with visibility, the analysis here will suggest that the erasure of women's needs is systematic, grounded in a complex array of media representations of the HIV pandemic, cultural beliefs, and research and policy paradigms which are deeply gender biased and not easily changed. This volume extends recent theoretical work in gender studies and relies primarily on close analysis of specific documents representative of several popular, research, and policy discourses.

In order to uncover the deeper gendering of contemporary discourses and to see how they are sustained and reformed as they shape research, representation, and policy in the HIV pandemic, it is necessary to step back, as much as possible, from assumptions about what woman *is*, and what social space she occupies. The general strategy of this book will be to explore how the issue of women has been raised in various aspects of the HIV pandemic, closely examining the underlying role of existing and evolving concepts of gender, including cases in which the most explicit concepts are about 'male' bodies and experience, leaving unspoken the experience of the 'other' bodies. Thus, the category 'woman' itself will be continually interrogated: how 'woman' is conceptualized — and by whom — strongly sets the terms for how HIV policy and education are formed for her, and how she is able to struggle against those whom she views as the source of her oppression.

This approach falls roughly into the category of what is called 'social construction' theory, now widely accepted as an appropriate framework for understanding the complex, mediated experience of the HIV epidemic. This approach assumes that social categories have been constructed through historical and social processes, and in such a way that the ideological and institutional interests served by a particular construct are erased and the categories appear to be natural. The task of the critic is to show how, and to what effect, such constructions arise and are used. While many academics are used to this approach, it is not necessarily intuitively plausible when applied to the conditions of women.

Few would explicitly argue that biology is destiny. Nevertheless, many would agree that while there are important historical and social differences in the category 'woman', there exists a bedrock of biological differences between men and women which must be respected, especially in the areas of reproduction, parenting and sexuality. Those who want to place great importance on pre-social factors like differences in biology view women's reproductive capacity as a source both of social power and of ongoing oppression and abuse. By contrast, a strict social constructionist position would object that even reproductive differences are made meaningful only in a social context, and the codifying linguistic procedures which accomplish this biological hierarchy must be analyzed, not adopted.

Clearly, both the idea that women are inherently biologically different than men and the idea that women are perceived as different than men only due to social constructions, arise in specific political contexts. Each idea has served to partially improve and partially limit the possibilities for those occupying the category 'woman' which arises from, and is dependent on, variations on these two basic premises. Abstract claims about women's needs are dependent on how women are defined, and these definitions and the prescriptions that flow from them come into conflict in policy, education, and research. Both biologically-based and social constructionist propositions inform aspects of AIDS policy and research, constituting the specific criteria for who will count as a 'woman' in a particular educational campaign, scientific study, or media report. For example, the US Centers for Disease Control uses the term 'partner of', subdivided into male and (predominantly) female, in its epidemiological counts. Highlighting 'her' partner status dovetails neatly with the larger cultural belief that 'nice' women's sexuality is passive. The infected bodies epidemiologically rendered as 'partners' connote passive receptors of HIV, quite a different image than the media's account of many of these same women as predatory 'prostitutes' who actively infect men. Likewise, the media's generic-sounding 'woman with AIDS' usually turns out to be black or hispanic, the partner of a drug injector, or a prostitute or drug injector herself. As detailed in Chapter Five, the occasional story of the white middle-class woman living with AIDS serves as the exception that proves the rule, simultaneously stoking women's fears and re-placing 'risk' outside the 'mainstream'. Thus, apparently substitutable terms have radically different connotative meanings across the media, epidemiology, and policy discourses.

The relative emphasis on women's biological difference versus her social similarity results in different, often strongly felt, beliefs about how to best 'help' women. For example, biologically-grounded systems separate woman as possessor of the womb from the aspects of women's bodies which enable sexual pleasure, counting as 'women' only those females who have and choose to use their childbearing capacity. Females who do not have children are ignored or even discriminated against — those who are no longer of 'childbearing age', lesbians (who, though such systems refuse to acknowledge it, might also bear children), or women who opt to use their bodies in other ways, i.e., for pleasure.

The systems which argue that women are the same as men may tend to minimize the different health needs of women or may be less active in providing protection for women who are subject to male violence or other systematic, gender-linked abuse. This second approach results in highlighting the social values or status of women, with little regard for biological differences in efficiency of HIV transmission or gender differences in the capacity to change risk-relevant behaviors.

It must be painfully clear to anyone trying to put women's issues on the agenda that this conflict between different (biologically) and same (socially) is not just a category problem, but the underlying paradox organizing research and policy: we are asking simultaneously for women to be treated as 'the same as' and 'different than' men. Policymakers respond with frustration: they interpret different claims about projects or policy as evidence of our confusion, or they divide women into two groups — those who are (like gay men) considered to be the cause of infection and those who need to be protected. This essentially racist and class-based separation of women is the same logic that has for two centuries characterized US public policies controlling women's sexuality and access to health care (Brandt, 1985; Rosenberg, 1962; Ehrenreich and Ehrenreich, 1971; Ehrenreich and English, 1973; Ehrenreich, Stollard and Sklar 1983)

A major reason for the failure to situate women in their various contexts is the heavy reliance of HIV policy and education on the ideas of risk groups and target groups. Given the focus on these related but not identical statistical concepts, women fade from view in HIV epidemiology for two reasons: first, considered by source of infection, women continuously appear to be statistically small in number, especially when broken down into gender subcategories of risk behavior groupings. Second, when 'targeted' by potential to become infected, the group 'partners of', despite containing a small number of men thought to have been infected by women, is so vague that it seems only to mean 'not men': male partners of men get their own category — 'homosexual' or 'bisexual'. 'Lesbians' are either heterosexualized or banished as 'other'. If a woman has had sex with a man since 1978, the Centers for Disease Control counts her as a 'partner', assigning anyone who insists that their infection is due to female-to-female transmission to the category 'other or unknown'. Epidemiological definitions of 'woman' continue to consider her a passive vessel or a moral pariah: women's risk is either decontextualized as a 'partnership' in a vast ill defined 'general public', or her body is constituted as the ground zero of sexual danger, as with 'prostitution'.

Powerful political and social institutions continue strongly to constrain AIDS work: emergency decisions and perceptions made early in the epidemic continue to shape the policy landscape, despite efforts to accommodate the growing reality that women are the fastest growing group of people acquiring HIV infection. However, activists and grass-roots organizers realize that they need these institutions' money and technical assistance, even while they pursue community-based projects in a language and style familiar to particular women. In order to explain programs or advocate changes in policy or law, it is necessary at least partially to adopt these institutions' concepts and premises.

Even the best intentioned administrator is hampered by the existing language available for discussing programs or policies. While highly critical of contemporary policy and media, the analysis here suggests that systemic practices and discourses rather than individual gatekeepers are responsible for the particular ways in which the HIV pandemic has been gendered. Chapter One will therefore review the early accounts of AIDS epidemiology and attempt to show how these produced a fatal educational strategy which pits 'deviants' (largely gay men and prostitutes, who need *policing*) against the 'general public' (largely middle class white women and adolescents, who need *protection*).

Chapter Two will examine studies of migration in order to show how the gender bias in the policy on which this form of research is predicated focuses attention on men and misunderstands the very women whom these men meet and with whom they form relationships as they migrate. Chapter Three explores the definitions used to understand women's situation in the epidemic and challenges the utility of identity-based concepts, controversial even in the gay communities which have asserted them, but which have become central to the AIDS policy and research paradigm.

Chapter Four will return to a more general discussion of the geographical and economic contexts which shape women's situation in the HIV pandemic, highlighting features which are broadly relevant to many categories of women. This will give an indication of the kinds of international policy affecting women that were in place when the HIV epidemic appeared. Chapter Five focuses on the discursive construction of women's risk by the US media during the first decade of the epidemic. Chapter Six offers a typology of existing programs and specific suggestions for conceptualizing policy and implementing projects in ways that are broadly applicable in a range of contexts, but maintain respect for cultural differences.

Readers will, I suspect, sometimes feel that I have given only partial treatment to the issues of women in the contexts they know best. My aim is not exhaustive treatment of any particular area in which women's concerns arise, but to show the existence and results of conceptual divergence. My goal is to provide a better overall picture of women's diverse situations and invite research and local coalition building, perhaps in areas which had not before seemed important or possible.

Chapter 1

Setting the Terms for an Epidemic

Emergent Syndrome: 1981–1985

Although the story of the early years of the epidemic has been told many times, it is important to recount it here because initial reports of the new syndrome not only set the terms for subsequent policy and planning, but also gendered as male the normative body affected by the syndrome, persistently constituting women as exceptions. It would be tempting to describe the first years as a time of great confusion and alarm, which would be rationalized and organized once the actual cause of AIDS was discovered. But the connotative meanings of those at risk for AIDS and the terms for researching and managing the epidemic were in place before scientists determined that a fragile virus (and still poorly understood co-factors), and not the lifestyle or behaviors of deviant individuals, was the cause of AIDS.

From 1981, with the publication of reports of the first cases of what would later be named AIDS, until late 1984, with the general *acceptance* that the newly discovered HTLV-III/LAV/ARV (renamed HIV in 1986) was the probable cause of AIDS, there were two dominant but competing explanations of AIDS: that there was a transmissible agent, and that immune system breakdown had resulted from overly taxing the body with sex and drugs. Although the former theory prevailed, the latter theory has lasted in the popular imagination as a 'rationale' lurking behind the kinds of people perceived to be at risk. (In 1993, scientists began to publicly admit that the immunologic explanation was also substantially accurate except that a virus, and not excesses of sex or drugs *per se*, inaugurated a complex immune system failure, making HIV a condition for, but not alone capable of, producing the clinical condition AIDS.)

In this early context of aetiological uncertainty, the media and folk accounts invoked the cultural narratives which seemed to most easily make sense of the medical evidence — those which could accommodate the possibility of either a transmissible agent *or* a defect in bodies or in lifestyles. Thus, the homophobic narrative of degeneracy could argue both that homosexuals 'recruit' (and will 'spread germs'), *and* that the homosexual lifestyle makes 'unnatural' impositions on the body which weaken it. Similarly, racist ideology which viewed black people as primitive could account for the initial cases among black people (largely Haitian and African immigrants to the US and Europe) as either a result of being too natural (and getting bitten by monkeys or, worse, having sex with them) or as incapable of adjusting to the physical rigors and discipline of modern life. And finally, the classic virgin/whore dichotomy enabled some women to be considered the victims, not of men, but of the lure other women's hypersexuality had for men.

These cultural narratives for understanding AIDS easily accommodated both overload theories and single agent theories of the cause of AIDS: risky behavior and risky people became synonymous, collapsing the process of infection into the fear of contact with people who are 'different' according to recycled stereotypes of otherness. In fact, the actual discovery of the virus made so little difference to the popular imagination that it has become increasingly common to encounter stories which describe early cases of people with AIDS intentionally infecting others. These apocryphal stories, of 'contagious' men and women who knowingly engaged in unsafe sex, attributed to individuals knowledge which they could not yet have had: those diagnosed with AIDS in the early years were already extremely ill and neither they nor those who were infected but not yet symptomatic had any way of knowing that they had a transmissible virus.

Certainly individuals had a range of responses to their clinical diagnosis with the new, little-understood disease, but it is crucial to remember that until the discovery of HIV (late 1983) and until widespread antibody testing was available (mid 1985), there was little popular consensus, even among researchers, about the dimensions or probability of sexual transmission. These early accounts — primarily featuring gay men and female sex workers — conflated the accusation of promiscuity with the stringent requirements for transmission, disregarding the extremely low efficiency of recipient ('passive') partners, regardless of gender, transmitting virus to the insertive ('active' and, of course, always male) partner. There continues to be debate about female-to-male transmission, which is much less efficient than male-to-female transmission, if indeed female-to-male transmission can be shown to be a major route of transmission at all.

The discovery of an aetiological agent established virology as the master medical discipline, pushing crucial immunological research aside. This double displacement of immunological ideas — into the popular unconscious, and out of the research race — was doubly fatal for women. The idea that people who have acquired HIV have done something excessive with their bodies continues to provide the foundation for many women's conviction that they are not at risk because they only engage in 'ordinary' (heterosexual) sex; it also leads to the continued emphasis on the danger of needle use at the expense of also promoting safe sex for women who inject *and* have intercourse with men.

The overemphasis on virological research also enabled scientists to discount the growing clinical perception that HIV disease was expressed differently in women. Since virology is chiefly a laboratory science concerned to isolate and act on a virus, the *body* of the person with HIV disappears, or is at best seen as an unfortunate complication in the quest to understand the natural history of the virus. To make matters even worse, women's bodies had long been treated as 'messy', subject to regular 'cycles' and to the intermittent cycle of pregnancy. In an important sense, therefore, the female body was the immunological body, a mess of countervailing forces always on the verge of exceeding the normal limits, unpredictable, always thwarting rational intervention by having uncontrollable side-effects.

Women in Epidemiological Accounts

Although it is commonly claimed that for the epidemic's first decade governments ignored women with AIDS, the picture of how women were related to the epidemic is more complex. A review of early accounts of the then emergent disease in the US epidemiological and medical literature suggest that women were early recognized as having the clinical disorder. But the significance of women as subjects of the disease was first mystified, then sensationalized, then marginalized by fragmenting women by behavioral categories which obscured the rapid increase in infections, especially in young women of color.

The Centers for Disease Control (CDC) referred to a woman with 'these two conditions [Kaposi's Sarcoma and *Pneumocystis carinii* pneumonia] in persons without known underlying disease' in early July, 1981 (*Morbidity and Mortality Weekly Report*, 1981a). Other cases in women were reported in August, 1981 (*MMWR*, 1981b), followed by another account which lists thirteen female cases and a 'proportion of heterosexuals [that] is higher than previously described' (*MMWR*, 1982). While a January 1983 issue (*MMWR*, 1983) describes two women, one with clinical AIDS, the second with lymphadenopathy, who were known to be sexual partners of men with AIDS, the column 'female' did not yet appear in summary epidemiologic counts. No full-scale analysis of women and AIDS appears in CDC reports until well after media accounts of the mid 1980s had presented sensational and bizarre accounts of women's risk for HIV. The next report to specifically address women concerned seroprevalence among 'prostitutes' (*MMWR*, 1987).

In fact, several distinct cultural notions of women were recruited to the media, policy, and research agendas, resulting in an overemphasis on female sex workers as vectors between the drug injection and 'mainstream' worlds, and underemphasis on the gendered dimensions of women's actual risk through sharing needles and through what came to be called 'ordinary' (penile-vaginal) intercourse. Highlighting race was a second, critical mode through which women were simultaneously dismissed and blamed. Sensational media attention to the research finding that women of color were over-represented in HIV and AIDS statistics, especially as sexual partners of infected men, shored up racist ideas that African-American and Latin sexuality were exotic and categorically different than 'white' (hetero)sexuality.

It was as much the appearance of women in the early epidemiology as it was gay activists' charges of homophobia that provoked the 1982 renaming of the new syndrome (originally

Gay Related Immune Deficiency — GRID) as Acquired Immune Deficiency Syndrome. But the initial association between AIDS and gay men was unshaken in the name change. Although little was known about the early cases among women, the media and policymakers suggested that women who acquired the 'gay' disease were themselves sexually deviant. Media and policymakers were early set on a course which associated women's risk with socially deviant behavior — even accounts of 'ordinary' women posed them as somehow exceptional, or as a 'later stage' of the epidemic in relation to the earlier cases in 'deviant' women. Policymakers' primary concern was with preventing crossover into the 'ordinary' heterosexual population. There was little concern to improve clinical understanding of AIDS in women, much less develop resources and educational strategies which could adequately address women's specific needs.

Clinical procedures for treating AIDS-related symptoms in men were initiated with the first cases, and a considerable amount of knowledge about variations in clinical presentation both regionally and by route of transmission was accumulated. However, variations by *gender* went largely unexplored, initially because the actual number of cases in women was considered too small for quantitative analysis. By the mid 1980s, there were as many cases of AIDS in women as there had been in men in the early stages of the epidemic when the original clinical protocols and research interests were defined. But now, it was said, the *percentage* of women as a function of the total cases was too low: scientific energies should go to the largest density of cases.

Worse yet, heavy emphasis on and debate over the construction of epidemiological categories by route of transmission overshadowed the increasing *clinical* perception that HIV progressed differently in women. Women were evenly split between route of transmission; about half had been sexual partners of infected men, and about half had shared needles with infected injectors. Since drug injection was viewed as ungendered, epidemiologists wondered whether, for purposes of defining routes of transmission, the latter group of women should be considered as any different than men infected through needle-sharing. Despite a continuing trickle of reports and case notes in the medical and social work literature, concern about the nature of women's clinical progress did not consolidate into a research enterprise until 1990, and only after considerable pressure from health workers internationally resulted in documentation of the degree to which women's opportunistic infections differed from men's. Only in 1993 did the Centers for Disease Control change the definition of AIDS and expand the list of HIV related illnesses to include the gynecological abnormalities and cancers which women had expressed or from which they had died. Thus, women were continually within epidemiologists' line of vision, but it took a decade to achieve official recognition of the uniqueness of their clinical and social experience of the epidemic.

The Birth of an Educational Strategy: Risk versus Population

The highly visible homophobia and racism and the sexism produced through considering women to be exceptions to a basic (but presumptively male) model were compounded by the theoretical paradigm most commonly employed in health education practices, producing nearly unshakeable categories describing what kind of education different groups of people should receive. While there are a dozen or so theories of health education commonly used in the US, most rely on one of two larger, general paradigms: decreasing risk for a health problem either by modifying the behavior of an entire population or by targeting only those believed to be at highest risk. Although, in practice, programs from different paradigms occur simulta- neously, they are usually *designed* with one paradigm in mind, depending on, first the epidemiological nature of a health problem, second, the perceived odiousness of the precaution required, and, third — importantly, though less often acknowledged — current attitudes toward those believed most likely to have or acquire the problem or disorder. Both the population-based and risk-based approaches recognize that individuals will be differentially affected by both the disease syndrome and the sought-after change, but differ in how they maximize disease prevention.

The population-wide strategy views risk as a continuum and assumes that many people are at some level of risk. An aggregate, population-wide decrease in the dangerous behavior or condition will also result in decrease among those most at risk. Critically, population-based programs perceive the health precaution or change to be uniformly healthy for everyone, and to be relatively simple and non-offensive to adopt.

Risk-focused strategies attempt to alert particular types of people to their special risk. Here, risk is viewed as virtually absolute: one either is or is not at risk. In addition, the proposed change is viewed as unfairly restrictive or burdensome or simply not useful enough to impose on those not clearly at risk.

Early AIDS Education: For 'Deviants' Only

From the moment that the emerging syndrome was linked with a homosexual practice in 1982, AIDS epidemiology and educational efforts generated from the public health service employed a risk-based approach. Rapidly changing social attitudes about sexuality and drug use rendered the notion of 'risk groups' highly equivocal because it relied on already labeled 'socially deviant subcultures' presumed to be virtually autonomous from the perceived mainstream population. Ironically, gay people's battle to reclaim once stigmatized social labels as a positive cultural identity meant that there was an uncomfortable convergence between groups' hard-won notions of 'community' and epidemiologists' labeling of 'risk groups'. Despite efforts among activists to shift the terminology from risk *groups* to risk *behaviors*, AIDS education information concerning risk *reduction* was directed almost exclusively toward gay men, and soon (though much less consistently and effectively) toward injecting drug users.

Although the risk-based approach was in motion in the US, little government *funding* was forthcoming. Public worries that promoting the less risky ways of engaging in stigmatized sexual and drug use practices would increase deviant behavior helped ensure the passage of specific bills like the Helms Amendment in the US, which denies funding to campaigns (and in some cases, to their sponsoring agency) which 'promote homosexuality and promiscuity' — a charge easily flung at explicit risk reduction materials and even at agencies that used public funds to buy condoms for free distribution. In effect, the decision by public health officials to use a risk-based approach in a climate of increasing social conservatism meant that little risk reduction information was ever produced and distributed by the US government. Risk-reduction education for those 'at risk' was considered 'obscene' and immoral; education for everyone else was considered unnecessary. The Centers for Disease Control Demonstration Projects, which survived largely by using complicated terminology ('men who have sex with men', 'people who exchange sex for money or drugs', 'hard to reach populations') and relegated restrictions on use of explicit material to their fine print, provided minuscule amounts of funding to a handful of nervously selected local projects. The vast majority of safe sex campaigns directed toward gay men were funded through private sources, usually individual donations from members of the gay community, and later, through Elizabeth Taylor's American Foundation for AIDS Research (AmFAR).

By the mid 1980s, it was evident that the 'general public' had developed problematic misperceptions about AIDS, especially regarding casual transmission. In response, a second wave of education was inaugurated, this time population-based education aimed at the 'general public', culminating in the controversial 1988 US Surgeon General's report. This wave of material largely assumed that while risk reduction knowledge was nice, the general population, never imagined to be at risk, should be educated about the impossibility of contracting HIV through casual or social contact. Although they had negative consequences in terms of risk-reduction targeting, pleas for compassion toward people living with AIDS helped establish a more positive atmosphere for legal battles in the mid 1980s which sought to classify HIV as a perceived handicap. This enabled people with HIV to claim discrimination under existing laws and, in some cases, forced the specific inclusion of HIV in city non-discrimination codes. But this also further entrenched the idea of 'risk groups' versus a 'general', if now more sympathetic, 'public'.

By the late 1980s, the apparent conflicts in the differing foci of population-based versus risk-based education had stabilized through the implicit constitution of exclusive positions for readers of educational messages. Figured most starkly in the concurrent messages, 'Anyone can get AIDS', 'You can't get AIDS [from casual contact]', and 'Change or else', AIDS information was targeted through stereotypical notions of whether the audience was at high or at low risk: it would have been difficult to *both* acknowledge one's potential for infection and view oneself as a good citizen *in relation to* people at risk of infection.

The first message was extremely ambiguous: the invocation of 'anyone' might dampen the association of HIV with deviancy, encouraging realistic assessment of personal risk by members of the 'general population' who indeed engaged in risk practices but did not identify with gay or drug use cultures; or the idea that the reader might be among 'anyone' might simply encourage more elaborate 'partner selection' strategies to sort out 'them'; or it might displace concerns about sex entirely, warning the general population members instead that they had better be nice because they would certainly soon know someone with AIDS.

The second message — 'You can't get AIDS from casual contact' — was intended to offset the broad panic which resulted in discrimination against people with AIDS. But encouraging toleration of, even altruism toward social deviants came at the cost of discouraging people from re-evaluating the potential for transmission in their own sexual practices. The third message, 'Change or else', invoked an unstated deviant practice and linked 'it' with virtually inevitable infection and death. This vague but frightening tactic discouraged those who were not already comfortable with their own homosexual practices (whether a dominant or minor aspect of their repertoire) from considering whether they ought to adopt 'safe sex' practices. Failing to specify *which* acts required changes allowed some people to rest comfortably in their perception that their activities were 'ordinary' and implicitly risk-free.

The problem faced by the consumer of education became less 'how do I avoid HIV?' than 'which campaign is meant for me?' The public health system educational programs targeted social stereotypes of HIV risk which merely repeated pre-existing stereotypes about class, race, age, and sexuality; AIDS education thereby became complicit in the ensuing systems of policing by portraying one group of people as needing to protect themselves from HIV and another as needing to protect themselves from the deviants subject to HIV. This economy of knowledge allowed the general public to press its claim to have a 'right to know' who is infected, while holding those 'at risk' to an obligation to ascertain and disclose their serostatus.

Separate Spheres, Opposite Strategies

This separation of educational efforts resulted in a quite dramatic and literal difference in the density of information available in the 'general' and 'subcultural' spheres. The very lack of information available in some spheres may actually reinforce the belief in lack of risk ('if it was important, they'd tell me about it'), while the multi-level and dense information within organized gay communities certainly contributes to a belief that risk reduction is important, even if not everyone always does it. In fact, different risk-reduction strategies were proposed in the two domains. The risk-reduction-information-sparse general public was encouraged to view risk as remote and to use avoidance tactics ('choose your partner carefully'), as suggested in the most extensively undertaken print campaign directed to the 'general public' in the US Surgeon General's Report (1988). For example, note the following advice offered in a section innocently entitled, 'What About Dating?':

> You are going to have to be careful about the person you become sexually involved with, making your own decision based on your own best judgement. That can be difficult.
>
> Has this person had any sexually transmitted diseases? How many people have they been to bed with? Have they experimented with drugs? All these are sensitive, but important, questions. But you have a personal responsibility to ask.

By contrast, the information produced within the risk-reduction-information-dense gay communities encouraged men to adopt routine use of condoms or simply avoid intercourse as a universal precaution. The introduction to the 1989 Dublin-based Gay Health Action Group's safe sex pamphlet is especially articulate, but not unusual in promoting universal precautions rather than partner selection as a strategy to reduce HIV transmission:

> The 'AIDS Crisis' does *not* mean that sex is a thing of the past. Sex can be safe. Much of what gay men have always done together has been 'safe', and has no risk of passing

the AIDS virus. It's simple to learn what's safe and what isn't.

Safer sex doesn't mean that we have to 'stick to one partner', or be afraid to start up with a new lover. . . . What matters is that we don't transmit the virus.

A 1989 New York Gay Men's Health Crisis pamphlet about HIV antibody testing expresses this same sentiment, advocating condom use even for those in monogamous couples who test seronegative:

Should I take the test so that I can stop practicing safer sex? If you and your partner use the test for this purpose, you both must remain absolutely monogamous, and continue to practice safer sex for at least a year before taking the test. This will ensure accuracy. If you are both HIV-negative, and stop practicing safer sex, you and your partner must continue to be absolutely monogamous. Unprotected sex with even one person may expose you and your partner to HIV infection. To avoid this risk, it is safest simply to continue practicing safer sex, even if you think that you are in a monogamous relationship.

The difference between gay-community-produced and public-health-produced approaches is even clearer if the above GMHC pamphlet is compared to a concurrent pamphlet produced by the City of New York 'For men who have sex with men', a phrase now commonly used in campaigns aimed at men outside the information-dense gay communities. Such men, here visually represented as African-American, are advised:

Here's what you can do:
If there is any chance that you or your partner might have the virus, use latex condoms (rubbers) whenever you have sex with another man or a woman.

Even if straight-identified 'men who have sex with men' succeed in identifying themselves as the target of this pamphlet, making condom use contingent on the conditional 'if' subtly promotes the avoidance strategy.

Each drift of HIV into new locales or new groups might have challenged the basic hypothesis that linked HIV to social or biological pathologies held to be intrinsic within an autonomous subpopulation. Instead, the original bifurcation of AIDS information target audiences into deviant and non-deviant set in motion a logic I have elsewhere called the 'queer paradigm' (Patton, 1985). Once perceptions of HIV risk were linked to social deviance, literally anyone, or any category of people deemed epidemiologically significant could be converted into nominal queers.

For example, Rock Hudson's death in 1985 should have undermined the belief in the existence of two separate spheres of risk. However, the perceived 'crossover' of HIV from the 'gay' to the 'heterosexual' 'community' — in fact, middle-class women — was explained by inventing another deviant: the 'shadowy bisexual', a creation which simultaneously highlighted women's *risk* and, by invoking partner selection as the route to 'safe sex', confounded risk *reduction* (how was she supposed to recognize him?). A page-one *New York Times* story, 'AIDS Specter for Women: The Bisexual Man' (changed in the inside heading to 'AIDS Specter for Women: The Shadowy Bisexual') (Nordheimer, 1987), describes this wave of AIDS panic:

> While bisexuals who are exposed during sexual relations with other men are one bridge on which the AIDS virus can cross from the high-risk homosexual population to infect heterosexual women, the greatest threat comes from intravenous drug users. . . .
>
> But numbers offer little consolation to the individual woman who fears that one miscalculation could be fatal, especially a middle-class woman who thinks the chance of contact with a drug addict using contaminated needles is remote. For this kind of woman, experts say, the figure of the male bisexual, cloaked in myth and his own secretiveness, has become the bogeyman of the late 1980s, casting a chill on past sexual encounters and prospective ones.

As long as policymakers and educators kept their focus on mainstream epidemiology within the US they could maintain the split between 'general public' and 'deviants'. But data from Africa persistently challenged the primacy of homosexual intercourse and needle-sharing as routes of HIV transmission. Racist Western beliefs that African sexuality is different, however, held off the call to re-evaluate the very basis of US educational strategies and public health policy. Indeed, even substantial numbers of AIDS cases, attributed to unprotected sex, among 'heterosexual' African Americans and Latinos did not break the original paradigm: these clusters of cases were likened to 'African AIDS', further distancing the white 'mainstream' from a sense of risk — or a sense of social responsibility.

Despite the massive official disavowal of women's risk in the epidemic, by 1986, women around the world were organizing *themselves*, particularly highlighting the universal aspects of women's experience of the epidemic. This universal discourse went a great distance in putting women in general on the global AIDS agenda, especially affecting policy in developing countries. But Western romanticization of the plight of third world women and demonization of economic development processes by post-colonial governments stalled serious evaluation of the differences in women's situations. Throughout the late 1980s, a handful of developing countries would generate innovative approaches to risk reduction by and HIV care for women, but these would have little effect on official US domestic programs. Though engaging in 'ordinary intercourse' and not considered 'deviants' the women in Africa were still considered 'other' to the 'ordinary women' in the US. Similarly, while homosexuals and sex workers in developing countries would be substantially indebted to strategies of people like them in developed countries, their governments viewed the local epidemics as being among 'ordinary' people who had nothing in common with or to learn from the 'deviants' from abroad.

Chapter Two explores some of the roots of the inability to understand similarities in sexuality across national borders and cultural differences. Migration studies carried out in response to the HIV pandemic provide a particularly dramatic example of the way in which underlying, unchallenged concepts of gender misdirect the very global research and policy paradigms which are supposed to provide adequate descriptions of and plans for people struggling to survive the new context of the HIV epidemic.

Chapter 2

The Gendered Geopolitics of Space

There are many, often intersecting, forms of population movement which make an individual's chances of contracting HIV
unpredictable, even if such movement produces sectors of greater
or lesser den ity on epidemiological maps. It is an accident of
history and of the geopolitics of global movement that HIV 'starts'
somewhere and 'goes' someplace else. But with the exception of the
export of infected blood products from developed to developing
countries, HIV has achieved its geographic mobility in the bodies
of infected people. Nevertheless, the heterogeneity which contemporary mobility creates allowed the media and governments to
revert to sheer xenophobia in their quest to confine HIV to
particular national borders, or rather, to keep it from slipping *in*.
Too much energy has gone into blaming individuals and countries, or trying to discover the 'original' locale of HIV. From the
identification of the first 'non-national' cases of AIDS within
European and US borders (respectively Zaireans in Belgium and
US Haitians in Miami and New York City), global epidemiology
and international relations, as research and policy enterprises, vied
for control over AIDS policy.

In the context of a new disease of epidemic proportions in
which the image of populations feared by the presumed 'mainstream' — homosexuals and black immigrants — initially loomed
large, the concerns of international relations initially won out over
the voice of global health policy. The blame-orientation
intensified because international relations has focused on the

nation, even while global health policy has recognized the fragility of geopolitical borders as blockades to communicable diseases. Recently, researchers have turned away from trying, implicitly, to trace the trail of blame and moved toward seeking to understand the dynamics underlying population movement in order to improve prevention education and care delivery. Nevertheless, the bulk of the research on mobility and the policy debates it informs continue to take the nation as the unit of space traversed.

The global epidemic of HIV has forced closer examination of international patterns of sexual behavior. Privileging the nation and the idea of development misses the reality that sexual norms and the symbolic meaning of sexual practices (even an identical act) are temporally and locally specific. The failure to theorize sexuality as malleable when it moves led researchers and policymakers to ignore important economic, political, and cultural factors which underlie mobility, supporting the temptation to deal with mobility problems through regulation of national borders. 'Homosexuality' was increasingly associated with the West by governments in developing countries, even while Anglo-European media and policymakers projected imagined exotic practices onto people in developing countries. In this context, discussions about migration and sexuality have been a massive outing:[1] an attempt to articulate migrants' 'other', non-home-state sexualities to the public space of national policy debates. But tourists and migrant laborers, indeed, anyone who has taken their sexuality across borders and cultures, know that crossing space creates new sexual personae. The varying styles of sexual performance discovered, invented, and transported are not linked within the individual's sexual unconscious, but dispersed throughout space, part, literally, of a journey.

The idea that there is something like sexual geography — for individuals and for cultures — should be obvious, but an anecdote will highlight the extent to which even the most ordinary sexual contracts can be spatially organized. About ten years ago a notoriously monogamous gay male friend of mine began regaling me with wild sex stories from his recent trip to the midwest. 'I thought you were monogamous', I said, fearing that his relationship was in jeopardy. 'I am', he said. 'It's Rt. 128 [the ring road around Boston, US] monogamy . . . I'm monogamous inside Rt. 128.' Couples and sexual networks around the world strike similar individual and collective bargains, and it is urgent that research and policy take into account the complex ways in which sexuality and gender are constituted in space.

Emerging Concerns with Migration

Shifting demographic patterns worldwide, but especially in developing countries experiencing heavy migration, have altered traditional gender and family relations with a range of negative effects for women. Various patterns of migration in and between developing and developed countries affect women either by increasing their risk of contracting HIV or by increasing the amount of care they will have to provide for family members with HIV-related illnesses and associated psychosocial adjustment problems. Although researchers were early aware of the role of migration in the dispersion of HIV little systematic study of HIV and mobility was conducted in the first five years of the epidemic: most media accounts relied on existing stereotypes about global movement. Research on migration converged with international law and policy debates in 1990; situating the International Conference on AIDS in San Francisco brought public criticism of the US, which refused to rescind its exclusion of HIV-antibody-positive entrants. An international scandal renewed in 1992 when the conference was at the last minute relocated from Boston to Amsterdam. But it was the rapid dispersion of HIV in Africa and Asia in the late 1980s and early 1990s which intensified interest in the social and epidemiological dimensions of migration in enabling the spread of HIV.

Although there is now a growing body of information on migration and mobility patterns as they affect and are affected by the HIV pandemic, rarely do this research or the national and international policy developed from it address the complex relationship between sexuality, gender and migration. The new, HIV-related research on migration implicitly accepts stereotypical notions that men are economic and sexual actors, while women are passive, virtual metaphors for the ground which male migration crosses. This results in bifurcation of research on mobility along gender lines. As traditionally conceived, research on migration largely concerns men. The primary area of research on women in the context of the HIV pandemic — sex work —

only hints at the mobility patterns of a narrowly conceived group, already a small subset of women. Thus, while there is a great deal of research about male truckers and male seasonal workers which presents a good description of their sexual patterns and identities, and while other studies have examined some of the kinds of women who might sell sexual services under these conditions, the actual interaction between women and truckers is virtually unstudied. Furthermore, education and policy concerning migrating men center on the 'proper' wives and partners the men leave behind. The reality that the women who work at truck stops as sex workers or hawkers also migrate and also have families situated in 'a home' elsewhere is apparently not considered. Mainstream research and policy have yet to move beyond the stereotyped perception that poor and uneducated women from the primordial countryside seep into mining camps or truck stops at the city's edge, where they are forced into a life of degradation and sin.

The underlying, but gendered, passive/active assumption in migration research doubles the already existing gendering of the object of study; the development schemes and legal structures which have emerged in most 'developing' countries result in employment and documentation practices which are implicitly gendered. Female migration is largely invisible, in part precisely because it is, in fact, substantially part of the illegal and undocumented economy of both developing and developed countries. By contrast, male migration, even when it defies immigration laws, is part of covert employment pacts between developed and developing countries, or is an explicit part of the economic plan in a developing country.

The rest of this chapter describes some specific examples of current research on migration, traditionally understood, emphasizing the ways in which assumptions about gender have made such work problematic. Also examined is research that does not take the nation as the central point of reference and which promises new understandings of sexuality on the move.[2] The rich possibilities for new paradigms suggest the urgent need to reconceptualize traditional approaches to mobility. Including other forms of systematic population movement will enable HIV planners to create sound policy and educational programs for people who experience their sexuality in multiple locations.[3]

Migration Studies

Traditionally-oriented HIV research and policy have usually equated the countryside or less cosmopolitan areas with low incidence and assumed that the most significant forms of migration are from rural to urban areas or from developing to developed countries. While these forms are important, overemphasizing 'migration' within developing countries and 'emigration' to developed countries obscures the role of economic, political, and cultural factors which cause and sustain regular patterns of movement, and leaves unnamed, and thus unstudied, forms of population shifts within developed countries and between developing countries.

Reconceptualizing structured and systematic population movements would highlight similarities between mobility patterns within 'developed' countries and between nations of the 'developed' and 'developing' worlds. In fact, focusing on mobility itself might lead researchers to choose study parameters other than the nation or development as the means of understanding how structured mobility affects sexuality. This chapter will select only a few ways of grouping studies that link sexuality and mobility: cyclical or permanent migration of males due to economic development plans; distant homosexualities; female outmigration for social or economic opportunity; migration of family units; 'gay' outmigration; and non-labor-related traveling.

There are other forms of patterned mobility which also result in individuals or groups existing in or between normatively distinct locales: these, too, could benefit from reconceptualization as forms of migration. For example, two forms of structured mobility related to US policy — Haitians confined to relocation camps while seeking asylum in the US and African American males victimized by structural unemployment patterns and social stigma resulting in cycles of imprisonment[4] — might profitably be compared. Because the causes of mobility in these two cases have substantially different symbolic meaning (national political strife versus domestic racism) they would typically be studied by different kinds of social scientists. But while the first case involves 'nations' and the second involves 'subcultures', both groups experience their sexuality in two locales which have different sexual norms. Haitian asylum-seekers are certainly aware that they are going to a new culture, while black prisoners may not think of their situation in that way. Creative planning for and with both these groups must include assessment of the meaning of living in two locales, a cultural reality that stems from larger political patterns rather than from individual decisions.

Mobility cannot be considered completely separately from the identity and status categories which those on the move may also occupy. The fact of mobility and social or status differences related to spaces may or may not be a conscious dimension of identity. For example, the ambitions of some tourists are framed precisely around the possibilities of finding greater sexual tolerance else-where, but so are the hopes of those who consider themselves permanent political refugees from areas of severe homophobic penalties. Men who consider themselves 'staunchly' heterosexual may not recognize the role of mobility in reframing their sexuality when they take up sexual practices with other men. In the first case, those who initiate their mobility because of sex and sexuality may have clear plans about how to enact their sexuality when they arrive at their destination. Those who do not (including women tourists who accidentally 'fall in love') may find themselves ill equipped to make sexual decisions. Men's presumption of social dominance over women may be dashed in homosexual situations, while women's hard won means of negotiating sex at home may go unrecognized in other settings.

To analyze events and situations in this way confronts some of the once comfortable assumptions about categories of mobility, and highlights the effects of mobility on sexuality instead of focusing on the relation of mobility to economic and legal problems. Thus, when the form of mobility called 'sex tourism' is addressed, it will be considered from the standpoint of the traveler. But it is also important to understand the mobility patterns of sex workers themselves, including the economic reasons for women's entry into this world of work as well as the loss of legal and social status which stem from engaging in sex work. Chapter Three will review some of the research and policy concerning sex work, examining on their own terms the sex workers who find 'sex tourists' among their clients. The review of these related groups of people has been divided in this way to suggest that sex while on vacation is not synonymous with 'sex tourism', especially for the woman traveler. This distinction is intentionally blurred here because it may be that the differences between purchased and 'found' sex, at least for the tourist, are not so sharp as they are for those who provide the sex.[5] Ideally, future studies of the relationship between sex and tourism will consider both sides of the commercial transaction, as well as describing the broader social and symbolic relations between less explicitly commercial bargains as these sexual-symbolic exchanges vary by gender.

Cyclical or Permanent Male Migration: The Classic Case

In many developing countries, male migration is a virtually permanent consequence of economic planning, resulting in gendered long-term demographic shifts in which men leave their partially dependent spouses and children in a home locale. Usually male migrants work for money: although they may make financial contributions to the extended family, and thus, indirectly to the home economy, this is at the price of their decreased contribution to subsistence agriculture or unpaid domestic and community tasks. This reallocation of men's labor cannot constitute a simple financial substitution, because in most developing countries the money economy and the subsistence economy are not fully integrated. The exchange value of goods produced — the money from cash crops or labor — does not equal the money required to buy the goods or services which would offset the labor lost when men are removed from the subsistence economy. Because these two economies are already gendered, with men increasingly integrated into the capitalized economy, the family *unit* may not experience class mobility, even though male workers are making money. Depending on the gender make-up of the cash-worker's extended family, with its support and its obligations, the 'cost' of replacing domestic and subsistence labor may be high, if it must be purchased in the cash economy, or low if it can be taken up by other family members shifting their workloads within the non-cash economy. In practice, shifting men into the capitalized economy simply results in increases in women's workload.

This gendered double economy is also present in the developed world, but is less visible since the transition to a capitalized economy structured around a nuclear family has been more gradual and is largely accomplished. Here, the stark and highly differentiated worlds of men's and women's work appear more subtly as wage differences and gender segmentation of job categories, with women concentrated in lower job strata. Thus, in the developed world, to the extent that men are expected to provide labor in the home, the removal of their labor to the wage economy can be offset; they may even be able to hire domestic workers, who will be either women or ethnic minority male laborers who are disadvantaged in the larger economy, for less than the value of the time they would lose providing domestic services for themselves. In both developing and developed countries this split economy makes women less economically viable than men.

The situation is especially volatile for women in developing countries because the shift to capital-based economies is still underway, and planners have often undervalued women's subsistence labor or not accounted for it in terms of its exchange value. Since this was the form labor took before capitalization, it is viewed as 'free'. The shift of male labor to the wage economy shifts the kind of production that occurs on arable lands and affects the percentage of labor devoted to subsistence, and women pick up the slack. These massive and relatively rapid economic changes make women more reliant on relatives, more responsible for local, usually non-cash crop agricultural production (in some countries, women have small, independent cash crops — generally, what is 'left over' rather than wholly different export crops), and more subject to cycles of economic depression since they frequently lack skills employable in the wage economy with which to supplement their own or their partner's failure to meet income or production expectations.

There are two material, geographically distinct effects of development plans which weigh differently on the gendered bodies that shuttle between them. The colonial and post-colonial shift toward geographically specific enterprises like mining have not only relocated male labor but have also resulted in increased food crop responsibilities for women, while decreasing their potential for earning real income from cash crops or cottage industry, with a concomitant loss in economic independence (Beoku-Betts, 1990, pp. 22–3). In countries that have initiated agricultural extension programs to ease the transition from subsistence-based agricultural economies to ones with substantial cash crops and exports, it is men who typically benefit. Whether they periodically migrate to mines or cities, or shift their farming to export crops, it is largely men who are enrolled in literacy, trade, employment, and agricultural extension programs. When new technologies are introduced, men generally control them, often increasing associated aspects of women's jobs. When labor-saving technologies are introduced for agricultural jobs previously allocated to women, men take over these tasks, leaving women to the most grinding, physically intensive activities. Pedal-operated threshing machines were introduced in Sierra Leone: men ran the machines on the cash crop farms, leaving women to thresh rice for domestic consumption by stamping on it. Ploughing technologies introduced in Sierra Leone decreased men's labor and dramatically increased the acreage of fields available for planting, but no technologies were introduced for weeding, harvesting, or clearing fields after harvest, jobs performed by women (Beoku-Betts, 1990, pp. 28–9)

Regardless of the local specificities of HIV seroprevalence rates, the economic shifts which promote male outmigration leave women locked into traditional roles in their home setting without recourse to the opportunities which have enabled men to find work elsewhere. Even if these patterns do not yet include significant numbers of returning infected male migrants, the epidemiological pattern combined with the increasing disenfranchisement of women suggests that when HIV arrives, women will be less educated generally, less economically independent, less likely to be in a position to ensure safer sex practices, and without the resources needed to cope successfully with the increased demands of caring for sick family members.

The Sacred Home

The dominant form of HIV and migration research examines this form of cyclical male migration from areas of supposed low incidence to areas of supposed high incidence. This pattern of migration is thought to increase men's risk of contracting HIV while away from a defined 'home' and thereby increase risk to 'their' wives or partners 'at home'. Little attention is given to the increased risk for the 'away' partners, women and sometimes men who are in contact with male migrants from widely dispersed geographic areas. In its starkest form, this work has framed migration-related risk as the transportation of HIV from commercial sex workers in cities, mining camps, or truck stops back to women in rural or semi-rural areas. This analysis is triply insensitive to gender, exaggerating the existing stigmatization of commercial sex workers, promoting the idea that rural women are ignorant and helpless victims of promiscuous males, and presuming that male migrants are inevitably driven to sex by the 'loneliness' of their situation and by uncontrollable sexual impulses. An early brochure explaining AIDS issues to journalists, produced by the World Health Organization, slips into precisely this understanding of sexuality when it describes one 'pattern' of HIV dispersion as 'the "army camp" pattern — possible wherever young men are together in large numbers away from home with some access to local women' (World Health Organization, 1989a, pp. 44).

Research with this kind of bias leads to intensified efforts to keep men from having sex while away, and has assumed that there is little to be achieved by promoting safe sex practices at home. For example, an otherwise useful pamphlet, from a series developed for African countries struggling to target education and allocate limited care resources, seems willing to sacrifice the female partners currently having sex with potentially infected men in favor of forcing a new sexual austerity:

> Condoms do have a significant — but limited — role in AIDS control in Africa, but promoting the use of condoms is a diversion from the central issue of *sexual behavior*. The practice of having multiple sexual partners is the main causal factor in the transmission of HIV in Africa. Promoting the use of condoms does not address this issue. It advocates a technical solution to a problem which can be addressed only through fundamental changes in social attitudes, values and behavior. (Strategies for Hope, 1989, p. 21)[6]

Reliance on the city/country dichotomy has led researchers to focus on the most visible examples of male mobility: truckers and male miners in Africa and migrant agricultural workers entering the US from Mexico. Early studies appear to have assumed that the women serving these men were already substantially infected and were the source of HIV transmission risk for migrant men. Researchers seem to have given little thought to the source of women's infection: typically enough, they seem to have been presumed always infected.

The traditional model relies on a 'boys-will-be-boys' approach to male sexuality, apparently assuming that truckers or miners are 'driven' to 'prostitutes' (or to each other) by the isolation of their situation. Despite ample description of the stability of migrants' 'away' relationships ('town wives' and 'regular customers'), HIV studies view the migrants either as promiscuous and as violating the norms of their home culture, or as single with decreased possibilities for achieving 'normal' marital relations because they migrate. Only recently have studies of migrating workers shifted their concern from the individual's pattern conceived as 'marital' and 'extramarital' sex, to interest in understanding the larger context of these sexual networks with the aim of promoting risk reduction, not just in the migrant male but among all partners in the several venues. This more recent model (developed initially by gay-sensitive researchers studying gay men's sexual culture) suggests that the various venues in which men have sexual relationships each have their own sexual mores, and it is the lack of coordinated interest in risk reduction across the whole network which results in 'at-home' women's apparent inability to achieve risk reduction.

Truckers

The Western media and much AIDS information material designed for use in developing countries represent the trucker as a major mode for the movement of HIV. Fortunately, the media stereotypes which construct the women at the truck stop as dangerous seem not to have been taken up by the truckers themselves. One of the rare studies (Orubuloye *et al.*, 1992, a study of Nigeria) that interviewed both truckers and women who sold sex, or who exchanged sex and other goods and services at the truck stops, found that both men and women were quite sexually active. However, the men made little distinction between 'at-home' girlfriends or wives and the women whom they paid for sex and domestic services at the truck stops where they regularly stayed. The study concluded that the pattern of sexual and economic relationships which characterized life in the truck stops was a deeply entrenched part of both the men's and the women's social life.

This is a significant reconceptualization of the truck stop from a place of unplanned encounter to a social/symbolic space with its own customs and mores. The 'life on the road' is recast from a transient space of male stop-over to a stable place of regulated sexual norms and daily reality: not an aberration from the 'real life' at home, but an alternative world. The distance between the lived experience of the truck stop and the media image of uncontrolled, desperate and dangerous sex engaged in there is in itself fatal, especially for the women who work in these venues. In a prevention discourse which requires identification of and with an extraordinary sexuality of 'risk', the men and women who people the truck stop are unlikely to view their relationships as out of the ordinary.

Of course, some health workers had already recognized the centrality of truck stop life for truckers and hawkers. A novel intervention with truckers suggests a future direction for work with men involved in this highly organized form of mobility. A recent project in Madras, India (Kumaresan *et al.*, 1992) established a health education booth at a major truck stop and used peer leaders to motivate other drivers to pick up information and accept STD and health referrals. A rest area with refreshments and music provided an informal environment in which to discuss health issues with other drivers and with counseling staff. An evaluation of the project revealed that the truckers were concerned with having been stigmatized as 'promiscuous'. As a result, confidentiality strongly affected their willingness to seek STD-related information and health care. This is similar to the study above: truck stop relationships are 'real life' and not furtive or shameful to the truckers.

Importantly, the evaluation showed that men from a wide range of locales outside Madras also stopped to get information and condoms and to relax. Like studies of bathhouses and other sexual venues associated with gay male culture, this study suggests that locales which have been stereotyped by outsiders as high in sexual activity and risk are symbolically meaningful places for participants, and can serve as excellent educational and referral sites. Future projects like this one should include the women who work at the truck stops, both as participants in the local sexual culture who are likely to be extremely knowledgeable about the sexual cultures of the diverse men they meet at the truck stop, but also as migrants who must also deal with men in their own 'home' settings.

Migration creates the opportunity not only for microbes to travel in bodies, but also for bodies to transport and encounter information. Hidden in the sexual behavior data of two Nigerian trucker studies (Orubuloye *et al.*, 1992; Gashau *et al.*, 1992) were incidental findings concerning media credibility: in general, the truckers preferred to receive information via radio. The preference for less local, more mobile information, and the interaction at the truck stop of men with access to a much wider variety of media suggests that truck stops in poor countries with limited media resources may be uniquely important sites of information exchange.

In the study by Gashau *et al.*, three-quarters of the truckers said that they believed that AIDS information services were inadequate and that they preferred to rely on international news, especially the radio. This finding has major implications for those designing programs because it suggests the opposite of the common-sense admonition to make information locally specific and 'culturally sensitive'. Here, international or national mass media appear to be more credible than locally designed, culturally-specific information: apparently, truckers view themselves as more sophisticated than the public which locally-generated information constructs.

Information directed to participants in differing forms of migration must take into account differences in class and education that may result in dramatic differences in access to and perceptions of information credibility. While the unskilled laborer who is the stereotypical migrant worker is likely to be disadvantaged by lower levels of education and may be less able to find linguistically compatible information than non-migrating workers in the same jobs, this is not necessarily true for all migrants. Other migrants, for example these truckers, may have very different patterns of access to information. Indeed, truckers, because of their age and stability of employment (respectively averaging 33 and 10.7 years in the study by Gashau *et al.*), occupy a powerful economic and social role. Their mobility has resulted in *greater* access to a wider range of information. If men like these are considered important sources of information, then *their* opinions and information may be valued above that of a local health service. This suggests that the information they distribute to other truckers, to the women they meet at truck stops, and in their home communities, could be at odds with or could reinforce locally-generated messages.

Educators who assess the beliefs of only those who stay permanently in a locale may overlook the significant role in information-giving of mobile men and women. If these men are a significant source of ideas about AIDS and HIV prevention for the women who serve these truck stops, and if their information is sound and credible, then the women who work at truck stops may have greater access to information about HIV than their non-migrating peers in small towns. In turn, educators would want to determine whether these women's views are credible to their non-sex-working friends. There is no reason to assume that the truck stop workers — largely unstudied, but often depicted as passive victims — are not already educators and prevention advocates in their home communities. Given that nearly all studies of HIV-related information now show high levels of knowledge about transmission, less knowledge about effective means of prevention, and even less effective implementation (very little condom use, folklore-based modes of partner discrimination), it seems crucial to assess the sources and credibility of varying types of information.

Distant Homosexualities

To date, most studies have focused on the potential for female-to-male transmission in the travel locale, and the potential this creates for male-to-female transmission 'at home'. Patterned migration also seems to engender homosexual subcultures in the 'away' location, with the possible result of creating two significantly different sexual cultures in which men operate, one of which is deeply socially stigmatized. A pre-AIDS-era study (Moodie, 1988) describes longstanding homosexual relations of male miners in South Africa, a set of domestic/sexual relations parallel to the 'town wife', a much described form of polygamous relationship engaged in by male migrant workers. Interestingly, however, Moodie's study suggested that intercourse was much less common in male/male, than in male/female sexual encounters. Thus, it is important to understand the behavioral repertoire which is part of the symbolic context of 'away' relations. However, the lack of a particular behavior in a particular locale should not be interpreted as evidence that men in that setting will never take up that behavior, an interpretation the South African Ministry of Mines made of Moodie's work in order to argue that interventions into 'homosexual' behaviors there were not necessary. Since sexuality is highly malleable, and given the cosmopolitan nature of many migrational settings, innovation may be more common, necessitating an ongoing understanding of sexual mores and practices in these places.

A recent study of Mexican male migrant workers suggested that men had adopted new sexual practices while in California, including male/male sex and oral and anal intercourse (Bronfman *et al.*, 1992). While male/male sex was not continued upon return to Mexico, men incorporated both anal and oral sex into their sexual repertoire with both casual and regular partners; some behaviors 'learned' while having sex with men were practiced with women upon return home. The interviews also suggest that recognition of the stigma attached to behaviors engaged in while migrating for work made it more difficult for the men to adopt safer techniques. The men were highly informed about HIV and HIV prevention, but because of the complex bi-cultural aspects of their sexual relationships at home and in the migration setting, it was difficult for them to acknowledge that they were engaging in high risk behaviors. Individuals may be most likely to assess personal risk from the most ideologically 'safe' identity.

Unlike the boys-will-be-boys stereotype which pervades most of the literature on the supposed deprivations of same-sex encampments thought to produce a compensatory homosexuality, both of these studies suggest that desire for affection and for domestic comfort are major features in the emergence of stable patterns of male/male sexual relations. The reluctance to create male/male relations upon return may have little to do with any innate preferability of heterosexual relations; it may rather, be a function of social sanctions in the original setting. Obviously, the greater the stigma attached to such alternate arrangements, the harder it will be to institute safer sex practices. Since most cultures value men by their ability to create a domestic and para-domestic 'home', but view homosexual relations as inappropriate, migrating men who construct these two forms of relationship will probably find it difficult to disclose their homosexual relations, even if they are acceptable in the migratory locale. But the availability of two worlds may sometimes result in men's drift away from their 'heterosexual' home; the Moodie study suggested that some men come to prefer their male/male relations and abandon or truncate their return to their heterosexual 'home'.

The extent to which migrant workers form relationships with men who are part of more openly gay communities is unknown. If these bonds prove strong, existing gay-community-based organizations need to modify their educational strategies to reflect the dual reality of the men they educate as homosexual. Likewise, migrant worker relief organizations need to understand the dual structure of sexual mores and sexual practices in which men exist, relieving the stigma attached to homosexual relationships and supporting the dual affective needs of migrant men. It must be recognized that while 'away' homosexual relationships may be similar in form to the 'town wives' with whom the same men may have relations, the power relations between men are significantly different than those between men and women, and the power relations between men who do and don't wish to disclose their homosexuality will also differ. Thus, as several studies of Anglo/European tourism in developing countries (discussed below) have suggested, the person perceived to be more culturally powerful may be perceived to be responsible for initiating and sustaining safer sex practices. For migrating men who have homosexual relations in the host country, it may seem that local residents are the authority on the need for safer sexual relations. Anglo/European gay men are more used to operating in a sexual negotiation environment approximating to equality; safer sex campaigns aimed at bisexual or homosexual men in areas that receive male migrant workers should stress the responsibility of the culturally dominant male. Further elaboration of the coherence of these male homosexual micro-cultures (which may or may not be 'secret') will afford better information on educating women in both the away and the home cultures about their role in evolving safer sex norms.

Migrating Women

The plight of women in developing countries migrating to cities has also been extensively discussed in the media and in international AIDS information literature, but this phenomenon has been much less studied in relation to the HIV pandemic. Unlike the descriptions of regular routes of male migration, women seem simply to appear in the cities. Part of the reason for this discrepancy in perception and the consequent lack of research is that female migration in the developing world is usually an unintended consequence of colonial and post-colonial development plans. Male migration is planned (if inappropriately understood) and part of the 'real' economy, while women drift out of unacknowledged roles in agriculture and into the undocumented economy of small-scale hawking, temporary unskilled employment, and sex work. It seems clear that some of the female sex workers in urban areas have come from rural areas, but there is so little information about their reasons for leaving, the course of their journey, and the networks they establish that it is difficult to know how to incorporate the women in these migrations into prevention education and health care planning.

Although the urban possibilities may finally be greater than those they find in their rural setting, women who migrate to urban areas are likely to find themselves at the bottom of the economic heap. There are few training programs for single women, and sex work may be the only means to achieve economic stability and generate capital to start small businesses. However, this work is stigmatized, competitive, and sometimes risky, requiring business and urban survival skills which some migrant women may lack. While 'training' is informally available through the community of sex workers, legal protection available to other workers is rarely extended to sex workers. Women engaged in less stigmatized work, such as sewing or selling goods, are also underpaid and are often denied or afraid to use social or medical services. Even in countries that have recognized the needs of migrants, fear of deportation or removal of their children prevent many women from making use of health care or training programs. Where the virtually permanent cycle of migration of males to work centers facilitates research, planning, and intervention, the also virtually permanent migration of women to the same areas has barely been studied.

Women who are engaged in commercial sex work may regularly migrate between cities due to general 'clean up' plans or because they have become known to the police. While the aggregate number of sex workers in an area may be stable, the actual total number of women involved is much higher because the women either move frequently, or move out of prostitution to be replaced by new workers. This means that studies of seroprevalence which show stable rates of infection may be obscuring an increasing number of new seroconversions.

Although urban life is harsh and competitive, many women prefer the relative independence and promise of opportunity it offers from the increasingly backbreaking rural life. Some women go to the city to gain additional training and skills, and become part of the professionalized 'modern' urban workforce (Kiereini, 1990, p. 7). Although they are relatively economically more viable and face less harassment than sex workers, their routes to finding partners — if desired — are different than those in traditional societies. Professional and semi-professional women in urban areas of developing countries face the dilemma that occurred in industrialized countries a century earlier with similar ambivalent results for women. While these women's salaries may cover their basic living expenses, they may not be able to afford luxuries or entertainment, and they may form bonds with men in order to gain access to the cultural diversions offered by the city. Here, 'dating' replaces the benefits of the traditional marriage.

The general decline in the importance of the family and traditional mores in urban cultures places women at greater risk, but also opens up sexual and marital bonds in ways that may benefit them. Urban cultures develop elaborate and class-marked modes of constituting domestic and sexual bargains: HIV and STD prevention programs should show an understanding of the complex calculus involved in urban survival for women, especially the different roles that commercialized and bartered sexual/domestic activities play in establishing status and economic viability for women.

Family and Large Scale Migration

Over the past half century, both Africa and Europe have seen large-scale migrations which include entire families. In these cases, women must provide emotional support to male partners who are under increased stress and must negotiate between old and new values. Adolescent and young women who are part of migrant families may wish to abandon 'traditional values' especially in regard to sexuality, but for a variety of legal, linguistic, religious, and cultural reasons cannot use the support and information systems which are available to their peers in the host country. In particular, adopting new gender roles and values about sexuality leaves young women and men with many questions which their families can no longer answer (Alma, 1986; Nejmi, 1986).

Several HIV-related studies are underway to assess the impact and needs of ethnic or linguistic minorities engaged in massive migrations. A Côte d'Ivoire study (Yelibi 1992) showed HIV-related knowledge to be significantly lower amongst those who had been part of the influx into Abidjan over the preceding thirty years, largely because their educational levels were substantially lower and because 18 per cent of them did not understand French, the major language used in the capital. Among the immigrant women, 38 per cent did not understand French, suggesting that women have even less access to information and are reliant on their more literate male partners or relatives.

Cultural Contact and Traditional Medicine

Unlike temporary or work-related mobility, large-scale migration has resulted in sustained and extensive contact between two or more cultures. In addition to the complex differences in sexual mores, there may be differences in disease nomenclature and in cultural systems explaining the cause, diagnosis, and treatment of illnesses[7] (Vernon, 1992, p. D426). Anthropologists have long been interested in the different names given to diseases by people in different cultures, but this interest was raised to the level of public fascination in the early years of the AIDS epidemic. In the early to mid 1980s, the Western media made a great fuss about the discovery that in Uganda, ordinary people had originally applied the name 'slim disease' to what was subsequently determined (in Western parlance) to be AIDS.

By the time of the AIDS epidemic, even the most remote traditional cultures had some experience with the Western medical concepts which figure so prominently in the research and discourse about HIV, and most traditional healing systems had already become hybrids, with some diseases considered appropriate for treatment by Western medicine. Remarkably enough, the pressure of the HIV pandemic, with the recognition of the significant role of mental health factors and of the embeddedness of 'risk behaviors' in highly culturally specific belief systems, has promoted a closer working relationship between traditional healers and their disease paradigms and 'doctors' and their Western paradigms (Pitt, 1990). Closer examination of traditional disease categorization systems suggests that 'Western' perceptions that HIV is a sexually transmitted disease have largely been incorporated into traditional medical systems, which also have categories for sexual diseases. In many cases, the prevention and treatment options proposed in the traditional nosologies are compatible with the categories and prescriptions of Western medicine. Although some curing concepts clearly do not jibe with current Western research, most of the prevention advice — including use of barrier methods — conforms to Western advice, even if the exact labeling and organization of healing categories is different.

In the early years of the epidemic, when 'Haitian voodoo' and obscure 'African' religious practices were promoted in the media as potential conduits for HIV and considered by educators and physicians to be *impediments* to HIV prevention. Recent years have seen greater plans for cooperation between Western and traditional medical practitioners, especially traditional medical practitioners (usually women) who have been the major sources of information for women regarding sexuality and childbearing. By the late 1980s, Western researchers were investigating a few 'traditional' substances in 'scientific' treatment trials.

This shift in Western attitudes about the relationship between traditional and Western medicine represents an important step away from the early presumption that traditional systems were mere antiquated mixtures of practical science and magical beliefs. Instead, medical anthropology has helped show that all concepts of health are culture-bound, and that successful international disease prevention requires validating and working within a variety of medical/social paradigms. It is not surprising that such cooperation would happen in relation to a disease for which Western medicine could not quickly find a vaccine or cure, and in which the routes of HIV transmission and prevention are perceived to be 'private' behaviors. The positive side of this partial leveling of power between traditional and Western medicine is the possibility that women will have greater control over prevention and greater involvement in development of care systems. However, Western medicine still dominates the research and clinical scene, and the small concessions to traditional healers can occur largely because their influence is in the domestic sphere which has always been seen as appropriate to women. Support of traditional healers is probably less a scientific concession to traditional medicine than it is a feminization of it.

Outmigration of Sexual Minorities

With the increasing visibility of alternative sexual lifestyles, especially the gay or bisexual lifestyles made visible through media interest in the HIV epidemic, the Western pattern of gay migration to major urban areas may become increasingly prevalent in developing countries. Little is known about the migration of sexual minorities; however, novels, case studies, and anecdotal reports of gay life in the international gay press suggest that a Euro-American-style 'gay identity' is now internationally available and being adopted by small numbers of men and women. The emergence of international gay and lesbian organizations and attempts to get organizations like Amnesty International and the European Council on Human Rights to protect lesbians and gay men worldwide suggest that the recent history of gay/lesbian community consolidation may increase. Along with the certain reality that some people who migrate for political and economic reasons will 'discover' their new environment to be more hospitable to their preferred sexual arrangement, intentional migration of gay people to more tolerable locales promises to have complex effects on the HIV epidemic. In Eastern Europe, Latin America, and Asia, the adoption of gay identity for previously unnamed homosexual social roles has promoted HIV organizing along the Euro-American activist model. But, at the same time, harassment of visible sexual minorities has increased, with uncertain effects in terms of mislabeling and stigmatizing those affected by HIV.

Travelers

The 1992 press coverage of HIV was dominated by apocalyptic and hysterically stereotypical accounts of sex tourism in Asia. Sex tourism is certainly a major phenomenon and could potentially account for transfer of HIV globally; however, to date, data indicting sex tourism is equivocal. Implicitly, sex tourism is thought of as people from more developed countries or settings going to less developed countries or settings with the intention of having sex. This general image obscures the range of relationships occurring between the participants. A series of phenomena occur under the now-sensationalized rubric of sex tourism, only some of which involve direct purchase of sex. These include general travel in which a male or female traveler seeks sex incidental to the trip, travel where a male or female traveler specifically but individually seeks sex, and organized tours where groups of travelers are taken to regular meeting places for the purposes of seeking sex.

A study of Canadian tourists in the Dominican Republic suggests that male tourists more often hire commercial sex workers for sex only, while female tourists have multi-faceted sexual relationships. Importantly, however, both men and women perceived themselves to be responsible for providing condoms (Herold *et al.*, 1992). A study of British and European travelers in London showed that those traveling to developing countries began new relationships with both local and European residents. Men had shorter relationships, but used condoms more frequently than women (Hawkes *et al.*, 1992). Thus, advice to travelers may need to reinforce the idea of condom use by male travelers, and find ways to empower women travelers to propose condom use in these probably intense, decontextualized situations.

Three studies of conventionally-defined sex tourists further complicate the picture. The first study, which examined Japanese male tourists in Bangkok, showed very high use of condoms during first encounters with particular commercial sex workers (Vorakiphokatorn and Cash, 1992). However, as has been suggested in a wide range of studies, condom use tended to decrease as familiarity with the partner increased. This is a particularly useful study because of the prevalence of condom use among Japanese, with 75 per cent of both males and females preferring condoms to surgical, intravaginal, intrauterine, or chemical techniques, and with nearly two-thirds of condom users supplementing condoms with abstinence during high fertility (Coleman, 1981, pp. 28–9). Despite the perception that cultures high in male dominance show low condom acceptance, Japanese men appear to accept condoms, even if women are the primary targets of marketing and sales. Studies of married Japanese couples suggest that condoms are not particularly liked, but are viewed as the most economical, easiest, and least potentially harmful form of contraception. In particular, the continual modification of condoms (size, shape, thinness, color, packaging) and the huge door-to-door sales by women to women, with the possibility of gaining advice on matters which are considered embarrassing to discuss in public, are all part of the cultural context which sustains Japanese men's and women's preference for condoms (Coleman, 1981, p. 37)

Two other studies compared gay and heterosexual sex tourists in Bali (Wirawan *et al.*, 1992) and Thailand (Wilke and Kleiber, 1992). Both suggest that gay male tourists are more likely to use condoms or engage in low-risk practices than are heterosexual male tourists. The rates of condom use in Bali were lower, which researchers suggested was related to the high level of alcohol consumption associated with commercial sex work there.

Compounding Infection with Dislocation

The HIV pandemic affects migrants in complex ways: in many cases, individual migrants who become sick return to their homes. This disperses the potential for HIV infection along migration routes, blurring the line between rural and urban disease patterns once observed in developing countries.

For countries, especially in Southern Africa, that are heavily economically dependent on the income of migrant laborers, illness among the male workforce or discrimination against workers may severely affect the national economy. Sick migrants who return home increase the care load of the people in the home country, a burden that falls most heavily on women since they provide the bulk of domestic and primary health care worldwide. Infected migrant women may be rejected from traditional support networks if they return home, both because their illness is not considered important compared to the needs of male relatives and because stereotypes about migrant women cast them as immoral, a view reinforced by the stigma already attached to AIDS.

The early recognition of AIDS in non-nationals in the US, Belgium, and France opened the doors to international travel restrictions. Exclusions are based largely on haphazard stereotypes about country of origin: India attempted to deport or exclude African students, the Soviet Union implemented compulsory testing of everyone staying for over three months, but was chiefly concerned about Americans and Angolans; the US used the AIDS panic to strengthen the case against admitting Haitians. But by 1990 as many as fifty-five countries, including the US, Canada, the United Kingdom and Australia, had imposed HIV-related travel restrictions, despite clear policy and human rights statements from the World Health Organization, the International Red Cross, the United Nations, and the Council of Europe decrying such restrictions (Cohen and Wiseberg 1990, pp. 36–7). The majority of these restrictions affect migrant workers and foreign students, but women are also particularly vulnerable because their legal status when crossing international borders is often contingent on their husbands or is undocumented, as in the considerable mobility of sex workers between countries in Southern Asia. Women are also more specifically affected when they are refugees seeking political asylum since they are especially subject to rape or forced sexual favors in exchange for entrance to refugee camps. In at least one case, a seropositive African woman was refused resettlement in the US for nearly three years (she was admitted to the US in 1992), even though her husband and children were admitted (Cohen and Wiseberg, 1990, p. 34).

Migration and HIV: Changing the Research and Policy Paradigms

As a global phenomenon, HIV is challenging traditional research and policy paradigms. International policy was complicated not only by national political differences, but by religious, social, and cultural differences concerning one of the most controversial areas of human life. Unfortunately, migration studies and international policy both focused heavily on the constituted nations and the flow of workers in and through formal economies. Though migration studies had begun to include sexuality as a feature of migrant life, international relations experts were hardly prepared to deal with sexuality as an international policy issue. Instead of recognizing the extent of human interrelations despite borders, the first decade of the HIV epidemic was a period of ill-considered international policy and unrealistic attempts to stop sexualities (often under the guise of nationalities) at the border. Researchers and policymakers in the 1990s are advocating the removal of barriers to mobility for people infected or presumed to be at risk for HIV. Some countries have designed and implemented complex and sensitive education and service projects for migrants in specific locales. But more attention to the complexities of sexual identity and evolving social norms is needed as, most importantly, are new research paradigms and concepts that do not assume that the nation is the most significant descriptor of sexual and social practices. Researchers must understand sexualities on the move as vibrant, exciting, sometimes dangerous and sometimes victimizing arrangements, and not as mere substitutes for something properly obtained at home.

Interventions are now needed which must not only combat border restrictions, but also confront the ways in which thinking of the nation obscures the realities of sexualities on the move. Policymakers and educators must understand that each locale and each form of sexual relationship has its own rules. Educational programs must shift from viewing sexuality as a property of individuals and instead prepare people for the complexities of cross-cultural interchanges characterized by relocation and return. Advice must prepare people on the move for decisionmaking in systems in which sex has different values and symbolic meanings and in which power and status will affect expected styles of sexual negotiation.

In an important sense, we are all migrants, encountering new rules and different meanings as we traverse our individual and collective sexual landscapes. Truly comprehensive approaches to safer sex will view all sexuality as the mingling of potentially different sexual cultures, requiring each of us to be educated and to educate others about the variety of possibilities for creating sexual identities and sexual practices which can stop the epidemic.

The next chapter will examine more closely the issues of labeling and social role categories articulated (or in the case of lesbians, left as a blank) by epidemiological and activist notions of identity and community.

Notes

1   The term 'outing' was coined in the late 1980s by gay activists in the US. Outing refers to the practice of publicly declaring someone else's sexuality, usually against their wishes.
2   I thank Benigno Sanchez for this term, which will also be the subtitle of a collection of essays on sexualities and borders, *Gay Diasporas: Sexualities on the Move*, edited by Cindy Patton and Benigno Sanchez, to be published by Duke University Press (Durham, NC).

3   The 1991 'AIDS and Mobility' report and plan produced by Aart Hendriks and the
    National Committee on AIDS Control of the Netherlands is an excellent example of
    mobility reimagined in order to understand the complex relations between national
    and political environments and a variety of forms of systematic movement — tourism,
    border crossing, work and sex work — and both sexuality and drug use as modes of
    exposure to HIV and other sexually transmitted diseases.

4   Billy Avery pointed out to me the similarities between poor African-American men's
    cyclical incarceration and the situation of migrants forced to move for economic
    reasons. In both cases, men leave a wide range of locations and end up in a single
    location — the mine or the prison — which has its own mores, and especially its own
    homosexual and drug subculture. The causes of African-American male underem-
    ployment and underdevelopment are well known and related to discrimination
    patterns which place all African-Americans in lower-paid jobs, but, because women
    can work in the undocumented private economy as domestic workers, males face even
    fewer opportunities for employment. Thus, prisons are a doubly gendered — and
    raced — phenomenon: they are gender-segregated, and the racial dimension of the
    prison population is related to gender-based employment patterns. This has several
    implications: first, that African American men are likely to operate in two very
    different sexual and drug use economies, that in prison and those in their home
    settings. The prison is very cosmopolitan, bringing together men from geographi-
    cally diverse areas. The stigma attached to both consensual and non-consensual
    homosexual sex in prison may make these men less likely to perceive themselves as
    addressed by education campaigns aimed at 'men who have sex with men'. In
    addition, their economic and social disadvantage within their non-prison localities
    may produce specific cults of masculinity which are not addressed in current
    programs aimed at 'heterosexuals' or at gay men. Although many US prisons now
    have good AIDS education programs (though few give inmates condoms), the reality
    that men are functioning in two distinct decisionmaking settings must be taken into
    account in programs both in prison and in the communities to which former
    prisoners are likely to return. Women prisoners are in a somewhat different situation,
    since theoretically and statistically, the female to female sexual practices they may
    engage in while incarcerated (and outside) generally afford less opportunity for viral
    transmission. Nevertheless, as I discovered in my own ethnographic work among
    women in methadone treatment, some of the best information women users received
    and remembered was that they received in prison. Again, women are being educated
    in and for two very different kinds of decisionmaking settings.

5   Regrouping sets of studies rather than accepting the labels of the scientists who have
    produced or organized them is a review procedure I call 'reading across the grain' of
    scientific reporting. While the strict comparability of studies may sometimes be lost
    (for example, sampling techniques may be different), unexpected similarities appear,
    and the naturalness of categories disappears. This method is especially profitable for
    planners and educators, potentially resulting in highly innovative planning that
    draws on research that might not have been reviewed if conventional categories had
    been maintained. For example, the extensive organizing and education by sex workers
    might be more easily transferred to projects for 'women' generally if the distinction
    between paid and unpaid sexual labor were dampened and the power relations
    between men and women highlighted. It might turn out that female sex workers, or
    segments of sex workers, have more collective experience with obtaining compliance
    with safe sex than have women who are not formally paid for having sex with men.

6   To their credit, the authors emphasize that condoms are not currently being supplied
    to African countries in sufficient supply to meet potential demand (Strategies for
    Hope, 1989, p. 21). However, this cannot be an excuse not to promote condom usage
    at all, since it is probably easier and quicker to increase condom supplies than to
    promote 'monogamy'. Indeed, the ease with which the lack-of-supply argument

becomes an excuse for not promoting condoms is based in the idea that 'in Africa, AIDS is a disease of poverty'. The role of social scientific research in supporting local educational campaigns is complex: for the most part, quantitative study can only identify broad patterns of behavior. Much of the 1980s research on 'African' sexual practices sought to identify a strange practice that could account for the statistical finding of a 1:2 or 1:1 male-to-female ratio of cases (thought to indicate female-to-male transmission, which had been largely ruled out in the US based on theories of viral passage through membranes and on the statistical finding of a 7:1 ratio of men to women in cases there). What statistics cannot show is the meaning of practices: how and why women seek and enforce risk-reducing practices, how and why they seek STD care. Future research on sexuality should be less concerned to find distinctive individual practices — there are unlikely to be many — and should instead describe the symbolic meanings surrounding the most risk-enhancing and common one: penile-vaginal and penile-anal intercourse without condom.

7 It would be wise to recall that the AIDS epidemic has seen continual clashes among Western research 'cultures' — chiefly between immunology and virology — which have also produced different beliefs even among Western scientists about the cause, diagnosis, and treatment of AIDS. To the Westerner, the differences within subdisciplines in Western medicine as a whole may seem less significant that those between Western medicine and indigenous systems taken individually. But this should not be interpreted as a matter of science versus non-science, rather as conflicts between explanatory systems which have locally rich meanings that provide hope and support for individuals who are ill as well as complex technical logics which are difficult to fully rationalize to those who are not trained in and socialized to a given healing art. 'Slim disease' seems stranger than CD4 counts to Westerners because we have come to *expect* our medicine to be expressed in symbolic mathematics and in names that have little to do with the physical experience or expression of a disease.

Chapter 3

Identity, Community, and 'Risk'

As described in Chapter One, Western activists have long struggled with epidemiologists and social scientists over the concepts of 'risk' and 'population'. In particular, gay men asserted the primacy of their 'community' and 'identity' while disputing the association of identity with practices. They argued that epidemiologists should focus on risk practices, even if changes to safe sex norms seemed easier to accomplish if gay men took on a positive identity that associated risk reduction with pride in self and community. Although the epidemiological categories only partially shifted to behavior-related terms, the 'identity' that had originally applied to gay men and the oppositional connotations of 'community' became central features in the social science research, education and policy paradigms. Researchers compared the practices of individuals who claimed 'identities' ('gay men') with those who didn't ('bisexual men'); 'education' was targeted at communities in order to help individuals 'identify' with risk reduction advice; and anti-discrimination policy protected those marked by 'identities' ('persons living with AIDS', too, garnered identity status). The presumption that the efforts to contain AIDS would be best organized around these specific notions of identity and community obscured the lived reality of four groups of women affected by and possibly infected with HIV.

Hidden within the epidemiological category 'partner of' or referred to in the media as 'heterosexual woman' it seems unlikely that women who might be described in either of these ways actually experience themselves as living in a community defined by their social relationships with men. Few heterosexual women were likely to 'identify' with risk reduction advice which had once been so strongly associated with 'deviance'. Chapter Five will detail the US media's construction of the 'ordinary woman' who was increasingly finding herself infected.

A second group of women, sex workers, was *in fact* 'partners of' men and formed oppositional communities not unlike those developed by gay men. However, policymakers were more concerned with sex workers as a source of infection to heterosexual men than as themselves 'at risk' *from* heterosexual men. Sex workers were 'targeted' through a highly discriminatory and moralistic stereotype, the connotations of which they did not, largely, claim for themselves: prostitutes. Policymakers did not consider the reality and strength of sex workers' communities to be an asset, but rather an impediment to the policing they viewed as necessary to halting transmission. Begrudgingly accepting lesbians and gay men, the media's use of terms such as 'heterosexual' and 'gay community' now referred to the collectivities of the two different directions of sexuality, not heterosexuality plied for profit.

Another group of women in developed countries was also obscured in the epidemiological category 'partner of' and lost in the generalized notion of a 'heterosexual community'. Female 'partners of' men with clotting disorders had formed a community around the centralized facilities for the management of hemophilia. Like 'prostitutes', these women lived in the 'heterosexual community', but their role, when it was visible in the media, was to symbolize the very essence of the traditional family. The wife and mother stood by her man, betrayed by the medical system, even if he infected her with HIV, even if she subsequently bore an infected child. The reality of her emotional burden was not well captured in the central paradigm which emphasized individual identity and affiliation with a community defined through sexuality.

Finally, lesbians who had been active in and partially articulated through the gay men's community during the AIDS epidemic were also obscured in epidemiological counts and considered exceptions to the central paradigm which links identity, community, and risk. Lesbians made and claimed their own name, but, in a paradigm in which 'identity' was supposed to suggest degree of risk, 'lesbian' was an ever-receding label since lesbians were considered by researchers and the media to be exempt from HIV. Identity and practice were confusing for 'lesbians' and for researchers: women who strongly identified with their 'lesbian community' were infected with HIV, but primarily through condomless intercourse with men, needle-sharing, and consumption of blood products. In the absence of a direct linkage between a specifically 'lesbian' behavior and a number of infections, researchers denied the 'risk' to 'lesbians' instead of recognizing that these women needed education and services specific to their small but separate communities. Lesbians would pose the ultimate contradiction between the idea of decreasing risk by reshaping community norms: the behaviors which form the major risk to women who identify as lesbians are largely not those which frame their sense of identity and community. Faced with a central paradigm that targeted education at practices through identity, and which had presumed female-to-female sex held no risk, both researchers and lesbians would have difficulty framing advice about needle-sharing and intercourse with men to lesbians without in effect saying that those they sought to educate were 'not real lesbians'.

'Prostitution'

After a decade of intensive research on seroprevalence rates among, and adoption of condoms by, women identified by researchers as 'prostitutes', it is now clear that sex work is often highly specialized and is extremely variable, with locally meaningful social codes and linguistic markers (de Caso *et al.*, 1992). Sexual bargains are not only specific to broadly defined cultures (say, the US versus Kenya), but vary by locale and form. Even within a city, seroprevalence and adoption of risk reduction are highly variable (Juarez *et al.*, 1992); however, the 'highest risk' venue of sex work in one city is not necessarily the 'highest risk' venue in others. But it is not something about a location or form of sex work which creates the zones of high seroprevalence identified by epidemiological mapping. Rather accidents of history bring HIV into a situated network. Dissemination depends on the precise details of sexual relationships between customers, workers, and their respective non-commercial partners, along with other factors like needle-sharing and medically-related blood transfusions.

Obviously, the use of condoms or the absence of intercourse from any one of the customer/client/non-commercial-partner network strongly affects the pattern of infection, but risk reduction and maintenance of low-risk or no-risk patterns are in part dependent on work-related variables and socioeconomic status (which are themselves related) (Bailey *et al.*, 1992). In addition, length of time and commitment to sex work (professional versus novice) affects the types of sex acts performed which also results in widely different degrees of HIV and other STD infections among sex workers. For complex reasons which are difficult to fully explain, Cohen *et al.* (1992) found that novices were more likely than professionals to be HIV-infected, but professionals more likely than novices to have syphilis. With both groups, HIV infection was more common in drug injectors than in non-injectors but this difference was not sufficient to account for differences in seroprevalence between the groups.

There are no doubt multiple factors underlying these gross quantitative findings, factors which are perhaps as specific as individual life histories: differences among partners and clients, in pleasure in or preference for particular sexual practices, in reasons for engaging in sex work, and in attitudes toward adopting 'safer' practices, which may require a more self-conscious commitment to the stigmatized social role of 'prostitute'. Shorter-term sex workers may be less inclined to view themselves as professionals who should adopt protective practices in order to stay in business over a long period of time. They may engage in sex work only intermittently and may not become incorporated into evolving norms for appropriate use of protective behaviors. By contrast, longer-term sex workers may have made more comprehensive decisions about electing to support themselves through sex work and may more clearly evaluate the risk to themselves of contracting STDs, as well as the risk to their business of refusing sex to customers who will not accept condoms or other protective measures.

More self-consciously professional sex workers may have more knowledge of and influence on safer sex norms. They may band together to require condoms and alter the accepted bargains on the street. Perceptions of professionalism may also affect clients' acceptance of condom use. In a recent German study, clients reported greater condom use in situations in which the sex worker was identified as a professional and the setting was less private. Public acknowledgment of prostitution and understanding of evolving sexual norms might alter clients' attitudes toward condom use. (Velten, 1992, p. D501).

The great variability among the women in these and other studies suggest that the category 'prostitute' is virtually incoherent, even though it is applied internationally, cross-culturally, and pan-historically (de Zalduondo, 1991; Pheterson, 1990). Pheterson has emphasized that the activities thought proper to the 'prostitute' are usually legally proscribed, her (or his) social status is stigmatized, and the stigma and legal status become linked. (Pheterson, 1990, p. 399). She argues that, in many societies, women who engage in the illegal activities defined as 'prostitution', even for a short period of time, acquire the social stigma and are not able to escape it, even when they stop the behaviors which are marked illegal.

Although prostitutes' rights advocates and anthropologists have long recognized the incoherence in the term 'prostitute', AIDS researchers and the media immediately adopted the term and its connotations as if they were unproblematic. The reasons why 'prostitute' was adopted are complicated, related to the immediate, empirical findings of early AIDS epidemiology (itself reliant on stereotypes), but equally reliant on broad and longstanding social attitudes.

Epidemiology is a science of categories: concerned to trace the origin and dispersion of unexpected medical phenomena, epidemiologists try to find descriptive categories by drawing on whatever ideas about existing social groupings seem useful in bringing a disease phenomenon under control. Given that the initial appearance of AIDS was among 'homosexual' men, a group perceived to be not only 'sexually deviant' but to constitute a tight and closed community, the appearance of HIV in *hetero*sexual men (most notably, the handful of cases identified by the Army among military men) required identification of an epidemiological vector. It was handy that those first 'heterosexual', non-drug-injecting men also reported contact with untraceable prostitutes in Germany. Many activists and researchers did not accept these men's accounts as evidence of female-to-male transmission (about which there continues to be considerable theoretical and epidemiological skepticism). But the concurrent discovery that some of the US women believed to have been infected through needle-sharing had also sold sex led the media and researchers to lazily conclude that 'prostitutes' were a *source* of risk *to* their paying male partners (though no one seems to have considered their husbands or boyfriends to be 'at risk'). In addition, early epidemiological reports from Africa suggested that the higher rates of HIV infection in women there were associated with something defined by researchers as 'prostitution'.

The underlying interest in the ensuing international research on 'prostitutes' was to describe how men who denied any other risk factor — 'heterosexual' men — might have become infected. Although used by the CDC and Red Cross as a donor deferral category from 1985 on, and later incorporated into HIV counseling and testing risk assessment protocols, the category 'prostitute' was not adopted to describe a group *at* risk, but only as a source *of* risk. Prostitutes emerged as the hysterical symbol of epidemiological crossover from a perceived nether world of sexual deviance into mainstream society. This misapplication of early epidemiology resulted in increased policing and harassment of women identified as 'prostitutes' in many locales around the world. Ironically, however, the same hysteria and misunderstanding to some extent created an opportunity for activists and researchers sensitive to the complexities surrounding sexuality to create projects and document the real risks to sex workers and the relatively low risk to their clients (at least, data suggest, in countries with higher levels of care for other STDs).

Although the category is incoherent, the education among sex workers has been partially successful in helping reduce their risk of infection. Evaluation of sex worker risk-reduction projects suggest that women who sell sex are more likely to adopt prevention measures (especially condom use or avoidance of intercourse) than are women who simply have sex in the context of recreation, love, or other socially condoned sexual arrangements. But the strong separation between sex for hire and sex for 'love' also results in a bifurcation of sex workers' risk reduction strategies. Women who sell sex are more likely to engage in prevention behaviors while having sex in the context of 'work' than in their domestic relationships. Several studies also show that condom use tapers off as a sex worker establishes a regular relationship with a client. Sex has a range of symbolic meanings and use of preventive measures also has symbolic meanings: apparently, the better one knows a partner — paying or not — the less appropriate it seems to enforce condom use. Like their non-professional peers, sex workers apparently do not experience themselves as 'at risk' when engaging in 'ordinary' (i.e., non-work) sex. This pattern follows precisely the advice to 'know your partner' promoted in the mainstream media and in public health brochures.

'Sex Work'? The Problem of Definitions

There have been many efforts to alter the stigma associated with sex work, and to promote better policy with regard to sex workers, most notably the shift toward the use of the term 'sex work'. This strategy originated in nineteenth- and twentieth-century Western feminists' attempts to improve the status of women generally by suggesting that the marital bargain and the commercial sex bargain are different only in that men's control of women's sexuality through marriage is legal. This approach focuses on the way in which social attitudes stigmatize one bargain, while forming a legal status and moral ideology to support the other. This argument has also proved useful when applied to women's situation in developing countries since women perceived by Westerners to be 'prostitutes' engage in a range of sex/affection barters to supplement their marriage or their other forms of income. However, these barters may or may not involve sex *per se*, and are frequently viewed as an extension of domestic services rather than as a separate commercial venture.

Thus, the term sex work is also problematic in the international context. While deconstructing the traditional negative connotations of prostitution, and signaling the labor issues involved, the term 'sex work' retains a Eurocentric bias. In the attempt to shift debate about bartered sex away from issues of morality and onto issues of labor, the term sex work privatizes sex by assuming that paid for sex is a commodified substitute for what properly happens at home. Organizing women as sex workers attempts to construct a notion of identity — as a worker — for individuals engaging in symbolically and practically disparate episodes of erotic commerce. Promoting the idea that bartering domestic services, including sex, is work requires introducing capitalist concepts of the split between domesticity and labor into cultures where such stark ideological and political divisions of labor either do not exist, or are a result of colonialist regimes.

'Sex work' does not fully reflect the experience of sex trade in developing nations, and probably also misunderstands the role and nature of sex trade in Europe and the US. For most men and women, trading sex and domestic favors is a transient activity. It may occur alongside stable sexual or domestic relations, or it may be a cyclical activity used to amass capital. In the Cameroon and other parts of West Africa, for example, rural women migrated to the cities and commonly own small beer houses which they capitalize through periodic sale of sexual favors. Alternatively, especially in Southern Africa where mining has resulted in massive and cyclical migration of men from the countryside, women (and sometimes men) who live near mining camps sell home-cooked meals and wash clothes, supplementing these cottage industries through trading sex with favorite customers. In the major Eastern African cities, such as Nairobi, where massive migrations have stabilized, a large class of women working in clerical or other low-level non-domestic jobs supplement their wages by trading companionship or sex for consumer goods, a practice known by names like 'going out'.

Renegotiation of domestic and sexual relations in countries experiencing intensive economic reorganization and massive migrations is extremely complex, and, as detailed in the last chapter, there is little research on the effects of migration on women in relation to HIV. Ideological rewriting of the history of modernization provides 'explanations' of the AIDS epidemic that collude with national morality campaigns instead of providing a basis for good advice. For example, literature and programs developed in Europe, but often implemented in conjunction with local Christian groups, invent for the African reader a bourgeois family which is represented as having been lost during the modernization process. Assuming that intercourse is the focal point of domestic relations, these programs associate condom use with the fracturing of African social systems and promote the bourgeois family as safe sex (Patton, 1992).

All redefinitions of social and medical categories are political, and impose new problems, even when they solve old ones. Though use of less stigmatizing terms is preferable, even the term 'sex work' fails to provide a broadly applicable concept for an array of culturally complex arrangements in which sex is systematically traded for benefits. Campaigns centered around 'workers' rights' in contexts in which the idea of a 'worker' as a distinct social and economic role is not present, or where female labor is not yet considered 'appropriate' (in cases, for example, where the difference in stigma between clerical work and sex work is minimal), may simply be incoherent to the women a project's organizers wish to reach. Emphasizing the economic dimension assumes an ideal case in which forms of 'pleasure' are purchased in clear transactions in which unit values are identifiable, and in which price has an autonomous meaning and is subject to market forces of supply and demand — but most forms of sex barter would seem to have situationally variable 'prices'; and the substitution of a second illegal commodity — drugs — into sex barter further complicates straightforward economic analogies.

Double Economy: Selling Sex, Buying Drugs

Recent studies in the US have tried to come to grips with the variability of the 'double economy' of sex and drugs, a situation so common that the Centers for Disease Control replaced the term 'prostitute' with the phrase 'people who trade sex for drugs or money'. This research strategy has made the mixed motives of participants clearer and shown that the co-inscription of sex and drugs places participants at risk of HIV transmission in widely differing ways. For example, professional sex workers prefer to receive payment in cash and, if they use drugs, prefer to buy drugs themselves. Indeed, men who try to pay for sex with drugs are suspect. At the other extreme are the young women and men whose lives now center around crack houses and who largely want to obtain drugs, but lack money to buy them and also lack the skills to enter sex work. The men with whom they barter sex for drugs are a resource.

The 'sex for drugs or money' nomenclature helps highlight the interrelationship between drug use and sex work. A complex economic negotiation occurs in the crack house and in other 'strolls' where drugs are substituted for money. The participants must quickly assign a 'value' to sex acts and to drugs and then come to an agreement about their exchange. Although the terms of exchange are specific to each transaction, the values are partly dependent on the costs to the respective partners of obtaining sex or drugs elsewhere. Especially with the high need to repeat drug use characteristic of crack, those buying drugs with sex may find it more convenient to stay in one place and perform repeated or prolonged 'cheap' sex acts (fellatio or hand jobs or sexual exhibition). But purely economic evaluation of these transactions obscures other major factors affecting whether those trading sex engage in high-risk practices. While the 'sex for drugs or money' nomenclature helps clarify the substitution aspects of the sex barter economy, it obscures the power relations which obtain in specific forms of exchange. From the standpoint of transmission, neither the relative transience, the number of partners, nor the quasi-commercial aspect of the exchange produces risk. The combined term also obscures the variable economic incentives in professional sex work, steady relationships in which drugs are part of the exchange, and the direct exchange of sex for drugs which characterizes crack culture. The relative autonomy afforded to women who buy their drugs with their own money is an important factor in their ability to pursue and achieve both drug- and sex-related risk reduction. Indeed, there seems to be a strong distinction made within the commercial sex world that trading sex for money holds more prestige, entails more autonomy and is safer than accepting drugs as even partial payment.[1]

However, gender differences in society at large, mirrored in sexual and domestic exchanges, are still underestimated in research on the role of sex and drug barters in the context of HIV risk-related behaviors. The exchange in a drug-using couple is considerably different than the exchange in a crack house; however, in both cases women maintain relationships with men because men are their means to obtain drugs. The reasons for failure to engage in risk reduction are also gendered, but quite different in these two cases. Introducing safe sex into a stable relationship is difficult under any circumstances, and long-term needle-sharers also have complex dynamics which needle cleaning may disrupt.[2] In the crack house, safe sex may simply not be sellable.

The insistence that it is the sexual exchange associated with drug acquisition which produces risk has led to confusion in crack studies, where the principal form of sex is fellatio, widely considered to be a low-risk activity. In the face of high rates of

HIV among young men and women who perform fellatio for crack, some researchers have hypothesized that the damage to gums and lips which result from the burns of crack pipes create more portals for HIV to enter the body. While this may account for some of these cases of HIV, other crack studies suggest that increased risk results equally from the relational patterns that have emerged alongside the actual exchange of sex for drugs. It appears that young women (and sometimes men) form relationships with older, drug injecting men who sell, but do not use crack. Thus, while these young people engage in very high frequency 'sex for drugs or money', it may be their 'steady' partners who place them at particular risk for HIV (Ratner, 1993).

Sexual Orientation versus Sexual Commerce

For the first decade of the epidemic, there was little research on clients of sex workers, in part because (male) researchers did not want to violate their privacy (though they were happy enough to violate the privacy of sex workers, who are at much greater risk of arrest) and in part because customers were thought to be difficult to contact. It may be true that few men acquire a social identity as 'john' in the way that workers acquire the identity 'prostitute'. At least in Anglo/European countries, hiring sex workers is seen as a quintessentially male privilege, not a source of oppositional identity (de Zalduondo, 1991, pp. 232–3).

But two studies, conducted in Atlanta (US) and in London, complicate social stereotypes about the presumed 'heterosexuality' of male clients who hire women for sex. The London study (Day *et al.*, 1992) showed that 37 per cent of men reported past sexual contact with men, with condom use highest in their commercial contacts. The Atlanta (Elifson *et al.*, 1992) study compared the ten year sexual history of clients of male and of female sex workers. Men who had initially been identified as clients of male sex workers had twice the rate of seroprevalence (37 per cent) as those who had initially been identified as clients of female sex workers (17 per cent). However, among the clients of male sex workers, 64 per cent had sex with both men and women, and among the clients of female sex workers, 43 per cent had sex with both men and women. In addition, 39 per cent of clients of male sex workers had also hired female sex workers, and 29 per cent of clients of female sex workers had also hired male sex workers.

These two studies suggest that paid or unpaid risk-relevant homosexual activity among clients may be an as yet poorly described route of HIV transmission *to* female sex workers. These findings raise serious questions about the past assumption that clients of male and of female sex workers are distinct populations, and that men identified as (non-injecting) clients of female sex workers were principally at risk from those sex workers (these studies seemed to take hiring a 'prostitute' as indisputable evidence of heterosexuality). In addition, condom campaigns which have focused primarily on heterosexual or on gay/bisexual men may have to reconsider the range of practices of the men they are trying to reach. Engaging in sex that is perceived to be 'commercial' may enable men to sustain one sexual identity while engaging in practices associated with another.

Instead of insisting on a universal definition of something like prostitution or sex work, it would benefit HIV planners concerned with women's needs to highlight the broad context of women's sexual, domestic, and economic relationships, rather than assuming that these are likely to intersect in any predictable way. While a casual review of research suggests that sex workers have been exhaustively studied, it is necessary to look more closely at the *forms* of research conducted. Epidemiological 'sentinel' studies, which hypothesize crude categories and then study groups thought likely to evidence HIV infection first, are quite different from the detailed and locally sensitive social science research needed to actually enable complex social actors to make changes toward lower-risk behaviors. Education based on findings from sentinel studies does little more than fill in the faces for a society's fantasies of risk, strengthening the association with stereotypical images of who is at risk, and resulting in misguided social policy and discrimination.

Hemophilia

If 'prostitutes' were the inevitable symbol of sexual excess and risk, women who were partners of men with coagulation disorders were cast as the stalwart wives and mothers who were coping with a disease that was not supposed to affect 'the family'. Shocked by the reality that products designed to save their lives were suddenly the source of a fatal disease, people with clotting disorders at first blamed the medical establishment and were bitter toward blood donors who were no longer perceived as altruists but as killers. Now laboring under a double stigma, men (and a much smaller number of women) with coagulation disorders, their activist groups and the agencies that served them were reluctant to be vocal about the extent of HIV infection among those who had used Factor VIII, a product designed for home use by those (mostly men) who had the most common form of coagulation disorder. And, until the late 1980s, the medical establishment, AIDS service groups, and the hemophilia service organizations themselves did not recognize the special needs of the women who were parents to or partners of infected men, and often themselves infected.

As with other stereotypes that circulated around AIDS, men with coagulation disorders, their wives and children were described in the media as otherwise nice, 'normal' families who were victimized by the disease whose source lay in deviant subcultures and the overly permissive society outside. 'Hemophiliac families' provided an image for the threat to the mainstream nuclear family of the disease of single, presumptively promiscuous, often homosexual individuals. Where the media produced alarmist figures on numbers of gay men infected in urban areas and decried their lack of behavior change, little was said about the high percentage of men with hemophilia A who were HIV infected, and who were also making only modest changes in the sexual practice that was sure to infect their female partners. If contracting HIV was seen as an inevitable consequence of being gay, a punishment for choosing a deviant lifestyle, people with coagulation disorders were also described as inevitably infected, punished for a defect in their bodies. Their female partners were described in heroic terms, and their infection through sex was supposed to be a badge of courage for standing by their men and families.

Programs or pamphlets directed toward women rarely took into account the specific situation of women who were partners of men (much less women) with clotting disorders. Unless they had been active in a hemophilia society or a treatment center, women who found themselves involved with men who had coagulation disorders were no better equipped to recognize the need for safe sex, much less negotiate it, than women in the supposedly HIV-free 'mainstream'.

Women had to help mediate the effects of the heavy social stereotypes which subject those who have coagulation disorders of varying severity to medical, employment, and social discrimination. Already isolated by the perceived need to hide their partners' or children's coagulation disorders, these women were further separated from potential support by the appearance of HIV and AIDS. Not only were such women often principally responsible for coping with the fluctuations in their partners' or children's medical and emotional state, but they were now also potentially infected with a communicable disease.

Public Image, Private Reality

Hemophilia, which affects approximately 20,000 people in the US, is the common name for a range of coagulation disorders in which lack of blood proteins results in delayed or incomplete coagulation. The public has dramatic misconceptions about the medical realities of coagulation disorders, most commonly fearing that 'hemophiliacs' will bleed at astounding rates. Coupled with the hysteria and misconceptions surrounding the communicability of AIDS, the fear that an HIV-infected worker or child would have a minor accident and gush infectious blood resulted in numerous cases of discrimination in the US, including the much publicized exclusion of Ryan White from school and the arson of the Ray family home.

But the real danger to the person with a coagulation disorder is not external bleeding, which is easily discovered and controlled, but internal bleeding, which is initially difficult to detect and becomes excruciatingly painful. Before advances in coagulation aids, joint damage was often so extreme that many people with moderate to severe forms of coagulation disorders were confined to wheelchairs by the time they reached adolescence. Individuals with severe forms of coagulation disorders had high mortality rates resulting from uncontrollable internal hemorrhage, including cerebral hemorrhage.

Before the development of home-use coagulation products, the treatment for bleeding episodes had been immobilization, ice packs, and transfusion with whole blood or plasma. In the mid 1960s, technological breakthroughs led to the development of products which enabled users to get a high concentration of coagulation factor in a lower volume of transfusion. This rapidly led to the development of home use products for less severe bleeding episodes. The most common disorder, hemophilia A, which ranges in severity, can now be treated through self-transfusion with a product called Factor VIII, made by combining hundreds of blood donations.

This unusual development of consumer-oriented products led to a radical transformation in the patient-doctor relationship: since people with coagulation disorders could now diagnose and treat their own bleeding episodes, what had once been viewed as a fatal disease was now a chronic and manageable disorder. Affected people born in the late 1950s and after were the first generation who could expect to manage their chronic condition and lead 'normal' lives. Unfortunately, this first generation of people with controlled coagulation disorders reached adulthood only to become infected with HIV through the very technology which had made them able to survive bleeding episodes.

About 90 per cent of people with severe hemophilia A were exposed to HIV before 1986, when donor screening was universally implemented and techniques for deactivating HIV in coagulation factor preparations were developed (Mason *et al.*, 1988, p. 971). Although the bulk of those infected through blood products were men, women who were their partners were at high risk for contracting HIV through sex: as many as 60 per cent of such sexual partners contracted HIV before 1986, when the new measures were effected. Women within the communities that had developed around hemophilia treatment centers experienced something like the assault on gay communities in early epicenters like New York, San Francisco, or Los Angeles: it took several years for communities and networks of people with coagulation disorders to reorganize medical, support, and education services after the recognition of extremely high rates of infection.

Care and Community

Unlike gay men, who had largely formed their community in opposition to government, people with the major forms of hemophilia formed a community under government auspices. Between 1968 and 1974, the federal government rationalized comprehensive care for coagulation disorders, raising the median age of death for people with coagulation disorders from 19.6 to 30.7 years (Mason *et al.*, 1988, p. 972) Impressed by the gains in the length and quality of life for people with coagulation disorders in comprehensive care situations, the public health service in 1975 established the Hemophilia Program under the Bureau of Maternal and Child Health. By the time of the HIV epidemic, comprehensive care centers were well established and were used by a majority of those with moderate to severe coagulation disorders. This centralization of care and training and the use of a family-centered model meant that after the initial shock of high rates of HIV infection among those at clinics, the National Hemophilia Society was able to recognize the needs of female (and to some extent male) partners of those they had been serving, including recognition of the special needs of women, children, and adolescents.

But the attempts to include partners and families of people with coagulation disorders did not always happen easily, and the need to consider infected partners strained the system. Coagulation disorders are genetically linked, not communicable, so there were predictable patterns of who might be affected — usually the male parent, or one or more children, but rarely the wife/mother. HIV affected female partners and children in new and initially unpredictable ways: women were now infected with HIV, and a child who was born unaffected by the father's coagulation disorder might now be infected with HIV. The centralized hemophilia centers, which had focused on making the (usually male) consumer less dependent on the medical system now had to shift toward integrating family not as supporters, but as persons themselves in need of direct care.

Several major issues emerged, which constitute in microcosm the experiences of women more generally. Relationships in which the man had coped well suddenly fell apart under renewed fears of mortality. Some men felt extreme guilt at the possibility that they had infected their partners and children.

63

Other men simply downplayed the risk, refused to be tested, or refused to adopt safer sexual practices. Women had to assume more responsibility for medical and psychological care even if they were also infected and ill. Many women reported that their relationships were quite traditional: introducing condoms or non-penetrative techniques into these sexual relationships was extremely challenging. In addition, although many consumers formed a supportive network through treatment centers, their female partners were often isolated, or knew only a few other women in their situation. Because hemophilia is so stigmatized and the partner's health insurance and jobs might be at risk, women maintained secrecy both about their partners' coagulation disorders and about their potential or known HIV-seropositive status.

Childbearing decisions loomed especially large. Because of the timing of medical advances, this first generation of adults whose hemophilia was well-managed were creating families at the point when the HIV epidemic appeared. For the heterosexual couple in which only the man was infected, the women who tried to conceive might not only possibly have a child infected with HIV, but was likely to become infected herself. The initial advice was to put off having children until more was known about the disease. By the late 1980s, 'waiting' was replaced by major social stigma against childbearing by those seropositive for HIV.

By the end of 1987, the US National Hemophilia Society had produced what is still one of the best pamphlets for heterosexuals coping with risk reduction. Concerned with 'psychosexual development' rather than abstinence, the non-judgmental pamphlet contained rare and sensitive advice about exploring non-intercourse modes of sexual intimacy — 'Do normal people really make love without having intercourse?' — and included information for teenagers and gay men.

Finally, women faced difficult decisions about what to tell their young children who were already HIV-infected. The medical consensus that patients *had* to be notified if they were found to be HIV-seropositive was designed with adults in mind. With seropositive children, there were different considerations: in the absence of any real possibilities of infecting others, parents wanted to consider whether the child could be trusted not to indiscriminantly tell others of their serostatus, whether they were able to understand the ambiguity of their medical situation, and whether physicians would be willing to provide prophylactic treatments to the child if the child had not been informed of his/her serostatus. Unlike social attitudes toward 'hemophilia', the public hysteria about AIDS meant that even very young schoolchildren had heard of the disease and had incorporated fears about it into their folklore. Thus, a seropositive child would have a difficult time staying 'in the closet' and would be subjected to the fears and childish understandings of the meaning of his/her diagnosis.

Activist analysis had hypothesized that traditional family relations and sharp division of emotion and domestic labor by gender would make female partners of men with HIV especially vulnerable. Safe sex might be difficult to achieve and the added burden might diminish such women's ability to care for themselves. The media portrayal of prostitutes as a *source* of risk led activists to put their efforts into decreasing repression of sex workers. Coupled with the image of the 'hemophiliac family' as the 'innocent victim' of the epidemic, the isolation and sexism faced by women who are partners of men with coagulation disorders was difficult to recognize. Oppressed through the quieter, more complex family relations which they both cherished and could not fully command, this group of 'women partners' felt little affinity with ideas of oppositional identities and were hard pressed to recreate communities that were not partly dominated by the medical system which mediated their care. While the National Hemophilia Society in the US, in the late 1980s, began to organize women using a self-help model, and while women who had contracted HIV through partners with coagulation disorders were prominent in the people living with AIDS movement, the majority of these women had to opt for playing out the drama the media had created for them.

Lesbians

If gay men's relation to HIV seemed ineluctably linked to a 'deviant' sexuality, and if heterosexual women's relation to HIV lay precisely in conforming to dominant ideas of their sexuality, lesbians' supposed exemption from HIV was apparently related to their distance from (reputedly) gay male 'promiscuity' and their break from the dominant sexual order. By the late 1980s, mainstream media articles on lesbians highlighted their nurturing, mainstream values, for example, their roles as middle-class professionals and mothers (*Newsweek*, 1990). Apparently, the strain feminism had put on the two-career, child-desiring heterosexual couple could be resolved by having two working mothers! Media accounts of the gay community's relation to HIV noted that lesbians appeared not to be susceptible to infection. Ironically, such articles proposed, lesbians visibly active in the AIDS movement and in health care were angels of mercy, Florence Nightingales who could move among both gay male and heterosexual female 'victims' without fear of contracting HIV.

Utopian ideas about lesbians' invulnerability rest on a compounding mistake about women's sexuality. The initial finding that women with AIDS had engaged in sexual intercourse with men who had AIDS was early used to assert their 'heterosexuality', even though researchers had apparently not questioned their identity or asked whether they had also had sex with women. 'Lesbians' were implicitly understood to be women who had not engaged in sexual risk practices, although the practice of male-to-female cunnilingus, the theoretical analog to at least one lesbian practice, was not much researched. After considerable pressure from clinicians and researchers who worked with HIV-infected lesbians, the Centers for Disease Control in the early 1990s began to investigate the sources of infection and seroprevalence among women who engaged in sex with women.

AIDS discourse had only partially separated risk practices from identities, confusing the role of identity in the formation of community responses with practices which were only partially shared by community members and were also enjoyed by individuals outside the self-formed communities. But where gay men's and lesbians' communities had been formed in relation to the same political forces and adopted similar political strategies, the confusion between community and identity played out in almost opposite ways.

Because AIDS emerged as a medical and media phenomenon strongly linked to gay community, early activists perceived the epidemic to be a dual assault — a disease affecting individuals and a political-medical intrusion affecting the fabric of gay community and, hence, gay survival. Early organizers refuted mainstream claims that gay men had 'caused' AIDS by citing lack of adequate sex education and STD care as the ultimate reasons for widespread transmission. Regardless of whether every gay man practiced safe sex, the earliest affected gay communities viewed safer sex as a political response to state mismanagement of sexual health, as something everyone should do or know how to do, and as empowering, even if perceived to be personally distasteful.

Early safe sex organizing related to a broad range of perceived sexual health care issues and served as a means for community-building. Coming directly on the heels of campaigns to prevent hepatitis B among gay men, early 'safe sex' pamphlets advocated total STD health awareness. By the late 1980s, however, this broader project had been narrowed to education largely about preventing HIV transmission. Safer sex guidelines for gay men were almost exclusively framed in reference to HIV, and safe sex was viewed largely as an individual behavioral problem.[3] While there may have been some logic to this shift (give information in relation to the most hazardous disease, rather than the universal problem of the condomless penis), the HIV-only strategy carried two problems. First, it seemed to contradict the advice in 'straight' sexual health pamphlets. Though these pamphlets had to compete with a larger media perception that also advocated condoms mainly to prevent HIV transmission, 'straight' pamphlets offered multiple rationales for condom use, including prevention of pregnancy and of all STDs. But second, the virtually sole association of condoms with HIV in gay men's pamphlets may have linked the *decision* to use condoms with the emotionally charged recognition of oneself and one's partner as at risk for a fatal disease. This probably undercut less dramatic calls to adopt condoms as a 'universal precaution'.

If men were getting mixed messages when addressed as potentially 'bisexual' in straight pamphlets, but 'gay' in gay pamphlets or the media, lesbians were in information vertigo. Targeted as 'women' by 'straight' pamphlets, as 'homosexual' by campaigns within gay communities, and admonished by the government to 'choose carefully', lesbians were no doubt familiar with but confused by three contradictory safe sex logics.

Although discussion by lesbians of their relation to HIV had occurred since the beginning of the epidemic, the idea of safe sex for lesbians entered public discussion in the gay and lesbian communities in 1986 when the Women's AIDS Network and the San Francisco AIDS Foundation produced the first widely available pamphlet for lesbians. Gay, lesbian, and feminist newspapers and magazines joined in the debate about what safe sex should mean for lesbians. Unfortunately, although the women's health and lesbian health movements had long been arguing for greater research on and community discussion about lesbian sexuality and its potential for STD transmission, the timing of these first national discussions of 'lesbian safe sex' meant that the idea of prevention almost immediately narrowed to a discussion of HIV transmission only.

The discussion was further complicated by another set of debates among lesbians: those concerning the prevalence and acceptability of 'fringe' sexual practices like sadomasochism. The controversy was compounded because s/m and other 'non-vanilla' lesbians were some of the early advocates of 'safe sex', especially the 'eroticization' of dental dams and latex gloves. The issue of bisexuality had emerged once again in the 1980s as women who had once thought of themselves as 'lesbians' either reclaimed the identity 'bisexual' or merely sometimes had sex with men, but continued to think of themselves as 'lesbian'. Discussions of safe sex were almost immediately confused with discussions of sexual diversity as lesbians fell prey to the broader cultural error of equating 'risk' and 'deviance', exacerbated by participants' own confusion and changing definitions of identity and practice.

The accusation by some lesbians that s/m practitioners had introduced HIV to the lesbian community echoed an accusation made by some gay men against men who practiced s/m and those who were active members of the bathhouse culture (which has no correlate in lesbian sexual culture). But while lesbians who advocated safe sex techniques and those critical of them proliferated positions on lesbians' risk and grew more divided, the major AIDS services organizations responded to the ambivalence about gay male s/m by producing safe sex pamphlets by and for members of the s/m community, inaugurating forums, and generally promoting a positive approach toward sexual diversity among their educators.[4] This is not to minimize the anger and division which occurred in the gay male communities, nor to overestimate the accommodation of diverse sexualities. However, gay men's institutions helped mediate (and sometimes exacerbate) these conflicts, while lesbians were left arguing without any means to coordinate discussion. Perhaps the early gay male ethos which viewed safer sex as community building and the consensus that HIV was otherwise a universal threat had made it possible for individuals with a range of sexual practices and beliefs to work together; or perhaps lesbians who were only just discovering the range and diversity of sexualities in their communities felt more different than alike.

Advocacy of safe sex was increasingly a line of demarcation: women who became associated with calls to safe sex, or who publicly claimed to use dental dams, were thought to have some suspect aspect to their sexual practices, and individual lesbians who raised the issue of safe sex and practiced it were immediately cast as the 'risky' partner. Thus, in contrast to the situation in the gay male community, where advocacy of safer sex carried no political risk, indeed, might be viewed as a positive contribution to community, advocating safe sex in the lesbian community quickly placed one in the camp of 'fringe' practitioner or political problem.

Some lesbians were openly agnostic about risk, but unwilling to use dental dams for oral sex. Paradoxically, this echoed the logic of straight men's principal objection to condoms, making an *implicit* evaluation of relative risk: change to awkward techniques could be put off until there was a clear and present danger. By contrast, when gay men discovered that condom use was sometimes difficult, or that giving up anal sex altogether was psychologically traumatic, educators quickly developed workshops and a rhetoric about 'eroticizing' safer sex, and 'mourning' the loss that safer sex sometimes necessitated. Similarly, programs designed for straight women enhanced their self-esteem, helped them practice methods of confidently saying 'no', and taught them techniques for erotically applying condoms to men.

But for many lesbians, the implausibility of much female-to-female transmission through oral or manual sex preempted major efforts to transform lesbian sexuality so that it accommodated alternative techniques.[5] Unlike heterosexual women, whose call for female controlled barrier methods resulted in the development of new products (however slowly, however crude the female condom, however problematic vaginal virucides), lesbians who pursued technical innovations were greeted as paranoid, ludicrous, envious of the attention gay men's sexuality had attracted, or masochistically willing to submit to practices which would shackle their sexuality.

Because the initial scientific paradigm virtually preempted research on lesbians and HIV, these political and community debates occurred largely in the absence of useful medical and clinical data. Lesbian activists — with a variety of positions on the issue of safe sex — suffered not only painful discussions within their communities, but hostility from researchers and program planners. Nevertheless, by the mid 1980s, virtually all calls to do more work on and for women from women-oriented health and HIV groups included a call to attend to lesbians' needs,[6] but exactly who the term 'lesbian' was meant to cover and exactly what should be done remained hazy. The case reports and statistics which could be gleaned from epidemiology and from theories of transmission suggested that the forms of sexual activity thought to occur between women carried little risk. While this might well prove true, it was a dangerous assumption to make in the early to mid 1980s when the only available data was based on conjecture and incoherently collected cases. Even early reports of a few cases in which women had apparently contracted HIV during sex with another woman were discounted by researchers: they argued that data collection was incomplete or that the women were lying. Even some AIDS activists quietly viewed the issue of female-to-female transmission as a political diversion and waste of researchers' time.

Despite being buried in the national methods of HIV accounting and despite the uncertainty about the risk of female-to-female transmission, an increasing number of women who identified as lesbians and were visible within lesbian communities were discovering that they were seropositive. With a few, highly disputed exceptions (O'Sullivan and Parmar, 1992), most appeared to have contracted HIV through needle sharing, condomless intercourse with men, or receipt of blood products. Clinicians and activists were now faced with actual seropositive lesbians — whatever their own route of transmission — who wanted to know how to pursue sex in their relationships with their female partners. With only shaky theoretical models of the biomechanics of female-to-female sexual transmission and no survey data describing how self-identified lesbians actually engaged in sex, activists guessed at what 'safe sex' might mean for lesbians.

There was considerable resistance among lesbians to early advice: to veteran AIDS activists, the resistance of the lesbian community and of researchers to the idea of studying female-to-female transmission was all too reminiscent of the resistance to studying gay male practices in the initial years of the epidemic. Some AIDS activists — and I include myself — believed that opening up the discussion of lesbian risk reduction was better than waiting until there were enough cases present for researchers to take female-to-female sexual transmission seriously enough to study it.

But studying female-to-female transmission was problematic to the politicized models of transmission invoked by both researchers and activists. In the absence of some indication that lesbians engaged in practices which differed somehow from manual or oral sex *between* the sexes, the medical evidence cited by researchers and activists to, respectively, discount 'heterosexual' cases and challenge the policing of sex workers could be put on shaky ground. Female-to-female transmission modeled women as transmitters, as did the dominant models which situated female 'prostitutes' as a critical transmission vector *to* men. The same epidemiologists who were impressed by the scant evidence which suggested that cunnilingus and 'deep kissing' might be routes of transmission between the sexes denied the possibility of female-to-female transmission through these same activities. Alternatively, the discovery of significant transmission between women might question the safety of practices which heterosexuals wanted to view as safe.

Activists, too, played loose with the meager data, citing studies which suggested that male to female transmission far outweighed female-to-male transmission in order to indict husbands and johns rather than 'prostitutes' as the likely transmitters of HIV, but ignoring such data when they wanted to maintain that female-to-female sex might allow for significant risk of HIV transmission. Paradoxically, evidence of transmission between women might undermine the arguments *against* overemphasis on women as potential HIV transmitters in the case of sex workers.

Lesbians and Drugs

If lesbians were invisible in, even excluded from, statistical data, they seemed consistently present in ethnographically-oriented

71

studies of drug culture and of sex work, many of which described or made reference to self-identified lesbians. These rich local accounts, however, did not jibe with debates among lesbians about their relationship to the epidemic. It seemed likely that most women who identified as lesbians and who were HIV-seropositive had acquired their infection through drug injection or through unprotected intercourse with men. To some, this disqualified their inclusion in the category 'lesbian'. For others, concerned to define a clearer picture of the broad social/sexual network of women, this increased concern that lesbian communities might be at a very early stage in the epidemiological curve.

In the early 1990s, researchers took a closer look at lesbians' sexual practices and drug use. Although their definitions of 'lesbian' vary, several studies suggest that women who have sex with women, or who identify as lesbian or bisexual, and who are drug injectors have almost twice the odds of being HIV infected as their peers who have sex with men only (Reardon *et al.*, 1992; Friedman *et al.*, 1992; Bevier *et al.*, 1992) The study by Bevier *et al.*, compared women who have sex with women with those who have sex exclusively with men, and found no evidence that the source of HIV infection in the seropositive lesbian or bisexual women was through female-to-female transmission. The most extensive review of lesbians diagnosed with AIDS (Chu *et al.*, 1990) also found no evidence of female-to-female sexual transmission, although the study cautions that more systematic prospective data is needed. However, while female-to-female transmission may be a statistically rare event, it is difficult to study because the majority of women considered so far have had multiple possible routes of exposure. Only occasionally and through detailed interview is it possible to ascertain *which* exposure has resulted in actual infection, and therefore which route is definitive. In addition, events which are likely to be statistical outliers — cases of seropositive women who had no other exposure to HIV — are difficult to find in large enough numbers to enable meaningful quantitative analysis.

The studies which find lesbian and bisexual drug injectors at higher risk of seropositivity pose several explanations for the finding, including the greater prevalence of sharing needles with gay men and the lack of targeted education. Female-to-female transmission alone could not account for the higher rates of seroprevalence, since male-to-female transmission and needle-sharing are still likely to be more efficient. While some cases of female-to-female sexual transmission may be hidden in the larger numbers — and this needs to be more aggressively studied — it seems most likely that identifying as lesbian or bisexual is a marker for social or informational factors which result in these women's failure to engage in risk reduction more generally. In my own ethnographic research at a methadone clinic, the tiny number of women who felt comfortable disclosing their sexual experiences with women reported several factors which might, on aggregate, account for the higher seropositivity of women who have sex with women.

For example, I conducted a lengthy open-ended interview in prison with a woman whom I had observed and interviewed earlier when she had been admitted into an emergency perinatal addiction programme. After an hour and a half, she identified herself as a 'lesbian'. She described her life as a cycle between frequent incarceration and unhappy relationships with men. She perceived herself to be a lesbian and considered her relationships with women while in prison to be positive, but upon release she 'tried to do what society wants me to do', and embarked on relationships with men, which had resulted in several unplanned pregnancies. Several other women I observed and interviewed also described positive relationships with women while in prison, but embarked on difficult relationships with men on release. Other 'lesbian-identified' clients seemed relatively isolated, with little support among drug users or lesbians. Compared to their heterosexually-identified peers, they lacked information on needle cleaning and were uncertain about their sexual-practice-related risk.

Two other studies that describe the sexual and drug use practices of women who self-identify as lesbian or bisexual also found that these women had, during the risk-relevant period of time, engaged in high-risk sexual practices with men (Hunter *et al.*, 1992; Iardino 1992). While both studies suggest that a significant number of women who identify as lesbian or bisexual engage in sex with both men and women over long periods of time, most of their sexual activity with males had occurred during their adolescence and early 20s. Iardino (1992) analyzed specific higher-risk behaviors and found two that might have implications for HIV risk level. First, women who had sex with both women and men engaged in both oral sex and penetration during menstruation much more frequently with other women than with men. This kind of difference in potentially risk-relevant sexual practices should be used to frame more detailed and discriminating epidemiological surveys. Second, while only 11 per cent reported drug injection, 27 per cent of these reported sharing with women only, 7 per cent sharing with men only, and 53 per cent sharing with both women and men. Given that women represent only a small percentage of the total number of people who inject drugs, the findings that a quarter of the women in this study share only with other women while only 7 per cent shared only with men suggest the existence of significant women-only drug injection groups.

Identity and Risk Reduction

Russell *et al.* (1992) assessed the attitudes of self-identified New York City lesbians toward modes of risk reduction. The sample, drawn from women at clubs and bars, appears to represent the more organized core lesbian community. While nearly two-thirds of these women believed that HIV could be transmitted between women during oral sex and 90 per cent engaged in the practice, only 19 per cent used dental dams or plastic wrap. About 40 per cent of the women said that condoms are the best method of safer sex in general, but since they associated condoms with sex with men, they viewed condoms as irrelevant to themselves. While it seems hopeful that women believe they should use condoms with men, this does not demonstrate that these women would actually use them, should they have sex with men. Indeed, the discrepancy between these women's belief in the risk of oral sex (whether or not it proves to be substantial) and their failure to take precautions suggests that perception of risk and use of risk reduction techniques are not necessarily positive correlates for these women. It may be that these women are engaged in partner selection practices and do not believe that any of their partners are or could be HIV-seropositive. In a context in which gay men's risks are so clearly documented and in which the epidemic is so obviously devastating, but in which their own risk is perceived as largely theoretical, lesbians are declining to systematically eliminate even the small risks they believe they face.

This chapter described the logic of identity and community which arose as part of gay men's resistance, then became the central paradigm through which researchers and media studied and represented the epidemic. But community and identity were problematic concepts for women: either researchers rejected women's claim to community or they allowed the concepts to obscure women's risk for contracting and clinical experience of HIV. The next chapter will shift focus to examine general features of women's situation which pre-existed the epidemic, but were exacerbated by it.

Notes

1   In my own ethnographic experience, many women remark that they would not go with a man who offered drugs. Others said that part of their job was to buy a certain amount of drugs for the client, which they would then also use. This did not affect their price, but was considered an additional service, in which their 'payment' for procuring the drugs was use of some of the drugs during the sex-for-money episode.

2   In my experience as an ethnographer in methadone clinics it appeared that introducing needle-cleaning was far easier for longstanding couples than introducing condoms. In addition, many older users already cleaned their works or maintained separate 'rigs': while this had decreased their risk of HIV transmission while injecting together, it created a false sense of security concerning occasions when either partner had shared with someone else. Like undisclosed sexual partners, drug using couples sometimes did not know about their partners' drug-using habits outside the relationship. In particular, women (and men being initiated into drug injection) who were dependent on men to obtain drugs or to inject them might not know how to perform needle hygiene if they injected with someone else.

3   There was always a current of community-building safer sex projects, including the 'Safe Company' project of the AIDS Action Community in Boston, that of Men Fighting AIDS in London, 'Rubber Fairies' projects in the Southern and Central US, and in the Tribes project in Sydney, Australia. Though sometimes funded through AIDS service organizations or the government, these projects always viewed themselves as oppositional and as having a broader community-building agenda.

4   For example, the various street/bushes/bar outreach projects educated outreach workers about the social and sexual dimensions of 'fringe' sexual practices and locales. I helped develop and for a year, provided this kind of training for the 'Safe Company' project in Boston. In addition, organizations with numbers of 'leathermen' among their caseloads quickly realized the need to give volunteers training related to diversity in the gay male community.

5   The community-building ethos was clearly present in a major portion of the early lesbian safe sex discussion. A number of the first interlocutors in the debates — including myself, Cindy Zegers and Beth Zemsky in Minneapolis, but also Denise Ribble in New York City and the women of ACT UP groups generally — in fact

had a background in gay male work and were explicit about the need to view lesbians' sexuality and discussions of safe sex in the broadest context. In all of our cases, the explicit political and community-building possibilities were raised continuously against objections that dental dams were problematic. The debate became lopsided and the sides missed each other, with the community-organizers appearing to ignore the problems individual women might be experiencing, and the anti-alarmism side apparently narrowing the issue to dental dams and epidemiological data about the incidence of female-to-female transmission. The community-building side, I think always saw the promotion of safer sex and caring for those infected as linked projects, while the anti-alarmist side seemed to have little to say about what to do about (and especially how to be the lover of) lesbians who in fact have HIV, regardless of how they contracted it.

6 For example, the statements by the International Working Group in Women and AIDS, active during the International Conferences on AIDS in Washington, Stockholm, and Montreal, always contained descriptions of the needs of lesbians and demand for their recognition as care providers and as infected women (Portis, 1989).

Chapter 4

Women's Health in a Global Perspective

Improved care and information delivery have resulted in increasing numbers of women around the world discovering that they have been infected with HIV, and more women are infected daily. Great variations in how HIV education and HIV antibody testing are administered, the availability of sexual and maternal/child health care, and social attitudes about HIV/AIDS, make it difficult to develop a single prototype program for educating, counseling, or providing medical and support services for HIV seropositive, at-risk or affected women. More fundamentally, cultural differences and the global perception that HIV is linked to socially unacceptable behaviors make women's routes to discovering and interpreting their serostatus highly variable. Moreover, media coverage of the epidemic in the West has promoted an image of women's risk that suggests that only extraordinary or deviant women are in danger. Women's perception of their need for information has been made contingent on understanding themselves as 'deviant'. However, women frequently recognize their potential for infection only after a male partner has become symptomatic with an HIV-related illness, or when a woman herself seeks perinatal care. Formal and informal processes to inform, support, and care for women with HIV have developed only recently in comparison to those for gay men in North America and Europe.

In response to increasing pressure to deal with the issue of women and AIDS, culminating in the designation of the Global Programme on AIDS' 1990 World AIDS Day, the World Health Assembly expressed its commitment to coping with AIDS by improving women's status throughout the world. This commitment built on the previous decade and a half of reports and policy recommendations which addressed women's status and needs in areas such as primary health care, anti-discrimination provisions and laws, economic development, maternal and child health, and literacy.

International health and development agencies had for some time recognized the link between women's health generally and women's social and economic status in the family, community, and society. In fact, women's health began to emerge as a keystone in plans for achieving health and development goals in developing countries, even though concern focused principally on women's roles as care providers and mothers.

The 1978 UNICEF/WHO International Conference on Primary Health Care, held in Alma-Ata in the then USSR was a milestone in establishing coordinated and evaluable international goals toward the achievement of 'Health for All by the Year 2000'. The Declaration of Alma-Ata, now a reference document and moral touchstone for progressive health planners, advocates greater local involvement in assessing and addressing health problems in communities, including food supply and nutrition, safe water and sanitation, maternal and child health (including family planning), immunization and prevention of local endemic disease, as well as coordinated planning linking community and national development. Although women's health is now used as a primary indicator of progress toward the health for all goal, there was no specific recognition of women's health needs in the original Alma-Ata plan, and women's health continues to be included principally under maternal and child health and family planning. While the implementation of some innovative primary health programs has enabled increased participation of and leadership by women in communities and at governmental levels, planners continue to overlook the negative affects of development on women's health (World Health Organization, 1987, 1988).

Two years before the Alma-Ata declaration, the United Nations had launched its Decade for Women (1976–1985) at a conference on women held in Mexico City. The midpoint re-evaluation conference, held in Copenhagen in 1980, linked the original 'Plan of Action' with the 'Health for All' goals to produce a forward-looking proposal that highlighted the complexity and interrelatedness of women's and countries' development processes, specifically linking women's legal equality and economic empowerment, control over their own bodies, and, especially, decreased violence with women's health issues. This proposal has served as a guideline for evaluation of local, national, and international initiatives designed to improve women's concrete health situations and their general social, political, economic and cultural status. International planning documents now frequently refer to these recommendations in the hope of recognizing and integrating the multiple ways in which the AIDS epidemic and its social impact complexly link individual health, discrimination, social and economic status and changing national and international policy.

While the particular needs of women and the forms of support available vary dramatically depending on economic, social, religious, governmental, and cultural factors, there are two virtually universal features of women's social experience which, while conflicting, have served as concepts for organizing women globally: women have local, often informal networks where much crucial folk knowledge about sexuality and social norms circulate; and the state, community, and society have an interest in women's childbearing capacity. Despite almost universal efforts to separate the state from private matters, counseling in the medical context and sex education/pregnancy advising in the social and family context cannot finally be separated, especially in the case of HIV. In societies without formal differentiations between community, 'scientific' medicine and centralized social services, learning, care, and decision-making regarding sexuality and reproduction occur among women. Such 'female matters' constitute the heart of the female infrastructure in such societies. Women in societies with 'scientific' medicine and centralized social services also have these networks; however, much of the control over sexuality and reproduction lies in the hands of professional gatekeepers.

In the HIV epidemic, the knowledge necessary for prevention is most easily disseminated through existing women's networks, while the technologies for disease detection and management are largely controlled by the state. Bridging the gap between women's ways of knowing and government/non-government organizations' ways of doing requires much translation. HIV-related programs for women represent a conjuncture between these forms of acknowledging women's interests. Adequate education, counseling, and care for women must bring together the informal women's networks with the clinics and HIV counseling and testing centers where most women discover their HIV status.

Until the late 1980s, there was little research on women in the context of HIV. Although it continues to be poorly coordinated, and often serves primarily to define gaps in research and services, there is now extensive epidemiological information and a considerable amount of social science research on women's situation underway. The latter focuses primarily on women's attitudes toward forms of sexual risk reduction (chiefly condom use and reduction in number of partners) and, to a lesser extent, on their perceptions of risk and their childbearing decisions. While HIV-seropositive and seronegative women are often compared in these studies, this only enables researchers to correlate attitudes with serostatus, and does not suggest what forms of counseling or social change might be most useful. Only a handful of studies assess psychological factors which might determine women's attitudes and concerns about risk reduction, and an even smaller number seek to identify social, psychological, and cultural reasons for childbearing decisions. The incorporation of qualitative and ethnographic studies to better detail the complexities of women's experience is beginning to provide insight into women's needs in the epidemic, but most research requires a great deal of reading between the lines to be useful to planners.

Given the structural and cultural impediments to developing health-related — especially HIV-related — programming, it is not surprising that there has been little formal evaluation of counseling programs' usefulness for women. Reporting data by gender suggests only how and to what extent women use existing programs: evaluation of programs designed for/by women are urgently needed. The lack of research initiatives in this area is exacerbated by the reality that most of the programs for women come from the grass roots and are difficult to contact or evaluate. Numerous authors have decried the lack of information on the myriad of local interventions, while activists and local providers have typically been unenthusiastic about ceding control over their programs to researchers. While the demand for 'no research without service' is worth backing, especially in the rapidly changing environment of the HIV epidemic, there are enough existing programs for women to more rigorously define their approaches, goals and criteria for success, and to try such programs in other settings. Evaluation is critical to expanding and supporting programs, but must not be driven by the anxieties of funding sources. New, mixed-method, and community-controlled forms of evaluation must be developed and should become as acceptable to planners and researchers as traditional styles of evaluation. This chapter will suggest the range of factors that need to be considered in designing programs, while Chapter 6 will propose concrete solutions and offer a beginning conceptual model for categorizing, comparing, and evaluating the strengths of existing projects.

Women's Status and Women's Health

The World Health Organization and its UN collaborating agencies have for over a decade recognized the intimate interrelationship between women's health and their social and cultural status. Both the end of the Decade of Women and the midpoint of the Health for All strategy show disappointingly little change in the status of women internationally (World Health Organization, 1985; House-Midamba, 1990). Although the status of women varies dramatically in specific locales around the world, when compared to male peers, women are virtually always less well educated, less well nourished, less politically active or powerful, and less economically viable. In most developing countries, the morbidity and mortality rate for females of all ages is higher, largely because women receive less health care, and receive it later in a medical syndrome (World Health Organization, 1985). In addition to less access to health care, lower levels of nutrition and calorie consumption result in higher morbidity and mortality for female children.

Women in some developed countries are now participating more actively in political and economic life. Legislation has given women greater legal recourse in cases of discrimination. However, women who are unable to make use of these legal changes are becoming even poorer, more than offsetting the gains of their more fortunate sisters. Even in developing countries, the minute gains women have made in terms of legal status and political participation are largely among the most elite women, who frequently do not share economic interests with other women.

In a detailed study of Kenyan women's advances during the Decade for Women, for example, House-Midamba found that women's participation is directly linked to their education, family background, class background, and participation in women's groups and activities, variables which are themselves interrelated, since education is related to family and class background (House-Midamba, 1990, p. 41). In addition, participation in women's groups enabled already elite women to form networks and develop skills in working in the interstices between government and non-government agencies. Although House-Midamba sees a small if solid level of participation by women elites, she cautions that the two most powerful women's non-governmental groups have been absorbed into the government in recent years. This may result in the loss of critical voices advocating for legal and social changes benefiting women (*ibid.*, p. 43). Women's movements in many other countries have witnessed similar loss of control over the articulation of political issues which they had raised as government agencies stepped in to fund things like rape crisis projects and battered women's shelters, but did not adopt the broader range of concerns evident in the feminist critiques which revealed the need for such programs.

The Africa Rights Monitor (1990) has also documented changes in women's status in Africa during the Decade for Women which suggest that the marginal increases in participation by women in government are usually in divisions or programs which are perceived to be of specific concern to women, such as 'community development, education, health, social welfare or women's affairs' (p. 49). This and other studies continue to decry the lack of indicators of women's status, from lack of statistical data on women's electoral participation to gender data on education and more sophisticated analysis of women's economic contributions.

The lack of progress toward women's equality and toward including women's specific health needs are particularly evident in the areas of literacy, maternal and child health, family planning, nutrition, economic status, and cultural attitudes. HIV and the accompanying social and economic crises are exacerbating these problems and creating new ones.

Literacy

Post-colonial development plans have emphasized population-wide literacy. However, observed increases are almost universally greater for men, whether measured by education obtained, or by people remaining with no education (Africa Rights Monitor, 1990). Increases in the education of women in the elite classes have occurred largely in humanities, teaching, and social sciences. Women continue to be excluded from the highest-paid and most prestigious technical and policy professions, areas which might enable them to participate more actively in planning and development processes.

In the past decades, with the increased concern with monitoring the health for all plans and plans for improving the status of women, female literacy has emerged as an important surrogate marker, not only for women's status, but for the health status of the country as a whole. Studies in developing countries and among the urban poor in developed countries suggest that level of female literacy, probably because it is predictive of options for economic independence from men, is a particularly accurate indicator of women's health status (World Health Organization, 1987). In addition, mothers' literacy correlates positively with children's health status (World Health Organization, 1985). While the reasons for these statistical phenomena are extremely complex and regionally variable, literacy in itself and as a surrogate marker for aggregate social status stands as an important indicator of women's status. While many countries have instituted special programs to improve women's literacy, the rationale for female literacy is as often linked to women's family obligations. While general increases in literacy have benefitted women, programs promoting female literacy do not necessarily have women's autonomy and equality in mind.

Women's generally lower level of literacy, especially in developing countries and among the urban poor, means that women are not easily reached by mass media campaigns and information brochures about AIDS/HIV. Lower literacy is also linked with less access to other channels of communication such as radio and television (de Bruyn, 1992). Even where women are semi-literate, the comparative difference with male peers means that they must often rely on male partners or male family members for information, including information about political developments and legal changes in women's rights. Men continue to be significant opinion-leaders in part because they have greater control over information (Africa Rights Monitor, 1990). When women with poor literacy skills migrate to another country, their language skills in that country may be even lower. Projects that aim to provide information in many different languages should also be aware that literacy skills in the first language may be low (Brockett, 1992).

Even in developed countries, where minimum literacy has reached close to secondary school levels, HIV-related prevention information may remain inaccessible. A US study of condom instructions, using three different measures of reading difficulty, found that of fourteen different sets of instructions found in the twenty-five major brands, only one required reading skills below that of a high school graduate, and most required the skills of a college student or college graduate (Richwald *et al.*, 1988). The authors of this report note that in 1980 (the date of the latest available data on US literacy rates) 13 per cent of white people and 21 per cent of black people had failed to complete high school, a measure which itself overestimates reading skills.

Maternal and Child Health

Women's mental and physical health have become of increasing concern in the past decades for several reasons. Women's role as primary producer of the next generation has become a major focus of international health and development efforts. Maternal health and skills are important because a woman's health status directly affects the birth weight and health status of infants, and because her skills and physical ability to nurture and care for children are strongly determinative of their future health and social possibilities. While the initial concern of these programs was child mortality, research in the late 1970s showed that maternal mortality in developing countries was at high levels. A summary of data gathered through 1983 showed half a million maternal deaths annually, with 494,000 of those in developing countries. Africa accounted for 150,000, Asia 308,000, and Latin America 34,000. In their most stark statistical display, this suggests that 99 per cent of maternal deaths occur in the countries contributing 86 per cent of total births (Royston and Lopez, 1987). Young age is an especially relevant risk factor in developing countries because early marriage is prevalent, and especially in subcontinental Asia and Africa, teenage maternity is common. But even in developed countries, maternal mortality rates for women under 15 are triple those for women between 20 and 24.

For culturally variable reasons, countries with low life expectancies also show higher infant mortality rates for males than females, but higher mortality rates between the ages of 1 and 14 for females than males (Waldron, 1987). When differences in cause of death are more closely analyzed, it appears that in settings where there is a strong preference for boys, greater mortality rates for female children reflect less nutrition, less medical care, and shortened child spacing (i.e., women have a next child sooner if the current birth is female). Although this is obviously a complex phenomenon, the observation of excess female mortality 'should be considered a warning signal for the probable existence of an important social problem, discrimination against girls'. Discrimination against girls, resulting in smaller size and chronic lower nutritional status, may work synergistically with maternal mortality when young girls then have children of their own. Data on highest levels of maternal mortality and on female child mortality point to the same cultural/economic patterns — those in subcontinental Asia and North Africa where the HIV epidemic has been slowest to manifest. The emergence of significant levels of HIV infection among women in these regions by the early 1990s suggests that women, doubly at risk from discrimination as girl children and again as mothers, will take an extremely heavy toll. These are the same areas where cervical cancer predominates: 77 per cent of all cervical cancers are diagnosed in developing countries with Africa as a whole, India, and Asia showing especially high rates (Stanley *et al.*, 1987). Cervical cancer in these regions is linked with early onset of sexual activity and with number of partners, probably because human papilloma virus, linked with increased risk of cancer, is sexually transmitted. Although cervical cancer is highly treatable if detected, only about 5 per cent of women in developing countries have access to screening, and these are usually lower-risk women. Most women are diagnosed in advanced stages when treatment is either ineffective or unavailable.

This cancer profile and the high rates of STDs in the same groups of women take on increased significance in the context of HIV. After considerable controversy among researchers, the Centers for Disease Control in 1993 changed both its definition for an AIDS diagnosis and its more detailed criteria for stages of HIV-related illness to include gynecological markers. This diagnostic and epidemiological monitoring system, which serves as the basis for AIDS and HIV-related diagnosis worldwide, now includes gynecological changes and disorders as early indicators of possible HIV infection and acknowledges their debilitating and fatal sequelae. However, the kinds of screening procedures which have made this connection possible are precisely those which are lacking in developing countries. Lack of cervical cancer screening with Pap smears, and poor STD detection and treatment, decrease overall gynecological health and make visual detection complicated. If the incorporation of gynecological symptoms into the HIV staging criteria has seemed of paramount importance to activists in developed countries, these are practically meaningless in the current medical systems in developing countries, where even routine gynecological examinations are rare and STD treatments are expensive. Nevertheless, from the standpoint of overall policy and resource development, these routine aspects of women's health care are essential for halting the worsening combination of maternal and gynecological disorders and the now fatal co-occurrence of HIV.

Obviously, it has been crucial to assess and improve technical facilities for maternal and child health; but it is not simply a matter of technically improving the care available to women. Women are most handicapped not by lack of sophisticated facilities to cope with complicated pregnancies or births, but in lack of access to basic primary health care and information. In many countries, self-examination and better use of traditional birth attendants could be far more useful than high-technology fetal monitoring.

In general, development plans overmedicalize pregnancy and childbirth to the detriment of women's health generally through the inappropriate deployment of resources, and by replacing potentially adaptable traditional female social practices with technological solutions controlled outside the community, and often by men (World Health Organization, 1985, p. 15). Women appear to use local programs that tap women's traditional support networks more often than they use clinical programs. If HIV information and counseling are only available in clinical settings or if they promote physicians as the most important 'source' of information, prevention will also be dangerously overmedicalized (Center for Women Policy Studies, 1990).

It is crucial to understand that throughout the world, it is women who provide the bulk of formal and informal maternal and child health care, information, and ethical decisionmaking support to each other. It may seem expedient to replace irrational or haphazard local systems for care and information-giving with standardized and professionalized programs and manuals. But as community health planners working in maternal and child health have learned, such efforts have failed and will continue to fail because they are not accepted locally, because they do not take into account the complexity of local social mores and customs which strongly affect overall health, and because the new social/health roles developed create new positions of power which tend to be assumed by those already in power. Programs aimed at improving women's health, but which displace women's traditional ways of providing care and information (even when these are technically problematic or unsystematic) with new, professionalized systems staffed by men or by women from other social classes disempower the very women who are the target of the health intervention. The most promising HIV education and counseling programs for women are those largely controlled by women of similar status to the women benefitting from the program.

Family Planning

Almost everywhere, women would prefer to have fewer children, spaced farther apart (World Health Organization, 1985). Ethical concerns about the utilization of abortion and of mechanical and chemical contraception must be assessed in the context of women's desire to conceive less often, as well as their reluctance to practice family planning due to fears of familial, spousal, or cultural repercussions. Thus, while tremendous energy has been invested in convincing women that they should practice family planning, it is social mores and male attitudes which have impeded family planning efforts most (World Health Organization, 1985). The media portray women who have one or more children after discovering their HIV infection as morally irresponsible, mentally unbalanced, or uncaring. However, when childbearing is the main role in which woman can attain self-esteem, even high risk pregnancies with significant odds of a negative outcome for the child may seem like a healthy and life-sustaining choice. Much of the early research on pregnancy and HIV was covertly aimed at preventing seropositive women from completing pregnancies. More recent studies have examined the features informing women's pregnancy decisions, demonstrating that knowledge of serostatus makes little overall difference in pregnancy decisions, and that social and cultural factors and not medical information largely determine women's decisions. One study of women who discovered their serostatus during a pregnancy found that while women were more likely to terminate the pregnancy during which they had discovered they were seropositive (and which entered them into the study) they were no more likely than seronegative women to opt for tubal ligation after that pregnancy, and there was no difference among women in their decisions to continue a subsequent pregnancy (Cowan *et al.*, 1990).

There has been considerable speculation that male partners or families have been major determinants of a woman's pregnancy decisions; however, a small interview-based study suggested that decisionmaking is extremely complex, possibly rooted in women's perception of their own agency, what is often termed 'locus of control'. A study of eleven women in the Northeast US examined the relationship between coping strategies, perceptions of self in decision making by women who discovered their serostatus while still within the time limit for a therapeutic abortion (Hutchinson and Kurth, 1991). While the women seemed isolated because the male partner was not seen as a source of support, this isolation was largely translated into a sense of agency and embattlement — 'just themselves and their children against the world' (Hutchinson and Kurth, 1991). As has been reported in other studies, women seemed more concerned about the health of their child than their own health, which Hutchinson and Kurth argue is not necessarily a self-esteem issue, since pediatric and maternal care are rarely well coordinated, leaving mothers in the position of having to choose between two poorly coordinated systems. Although only three of the eleven women chose to terminate their pregnancies, all expressed a desire to have the option. Religious and other beliefs proved important in the decisionmaking process, but the study emphasizes that a process of decisionmaking occurred and the possibility of choosing made the final decision more emotionally acceptable. Like other studies of this kind, the seropositive women, many of whom were from disadvantaged inner-city settings, saw motherhood as a central focus of their life, not only as a source of happiness, but as a reminder of the importance of staying off drugs and being involved in the social world (Pivnick, 1991).

Another study (Holman *et al.*, 1989) emphasized the stress placed on women by their decisions to disclose their status to their male partners: only twenty-seven of the eighty-two subjects who learned their serostatus after becoming pregnant received their test results within the time limit for a therapeutic abortion. Of these women, four chose to abort, and a fifth sought abortion but could not find an outpatient clinic that would take a methadone-maintained person at her dose level. The woman would not accept an inpatient admission because she feared her family would learn about the abortion. Most women informed their steady partners within two months, and only two relationships appeared to break up as a result, but several relationships broke up for other reasons, such as continued drug use.

Finally, the desire to have and raise children (albeit on her own schedule) and the fear of losing children to social service officials place the HIV seropositive woman in a difficult position: she knows that she and her child need special health care, but she is reluctant to go to the clinic because she fears her child will be taken away.

Malnutrition

Not only are there nutritional differences between male and female children, but adult women in poorer countries and urban areas also experience lower nutritional status than their male peers (World Health Organization, 1987). This results in generally lower health status and particularly worsens the anemia common among women of childbearing age (Royston and

Armstrong, 1989). Malnutrition and anemia decrease women's ability to perform their jobs due to fatigue and greater susceptibility to other illnesses, and increase the possibilities of death during childbearing (World Health Organization, 1990). In sections of the world heavily dependent on female agricultural labor, HIV may exacerbate existing nutritional deficiencies and affect overall food production, again increasing women's workload.

Furthermore, the solution to maternal anemia in much of Africa has been whole blood transfusion, now a potential source of HIV infection. According to some studies, the significance of transfusion-related HIV infection for women in countries where transfusion is a common treatment for anemia, and for low-income women who may suffer increased childbirth complications requiring transfusion, has been missed because women requiring transfusion–s in such cases will have been 'partners of' potentially infected men (Fleming, 1988).

Early motherhood and malnutrition also interact hazardously for young women. In addition to complications arising from the fact that her pelvic cavity is not fully developed, sharing nutrition with the developing fetus decreases the nutrients available for the young woman to complete her own growth. The woman and child suffer from the general effects of malnutrition, and neither has sufficient calories or nutrients to develop properly (World Health Organization, 1989b).

If the physical effects of early childbearing are roughly universal, the social effects are highly specific. The patterns of young childbearing are complex, with rates highest in Africa and lowest in Europe and Asia, with the US and Latin America in between, but these patterns must be examined in their cultural context. In traditional societies, the demands for emotional and economic support as well as instruction in childrearing may be partly lessened by the existence of extended family networks. Although France and the US have considerably different rates of birth by women under age 20 (18 and 53 per 1000), in both countries a significant number of those women were unmarried (51 per cent and 38 per cent respectively). Young childbearers are likely to be poor, possibly alienated from family networks, and more reliant on social welfare systems which may discriminate on the basis of marital status. This pattern is increasing in developing countries: studies of marriage patterns suggest that while age of marriage is increasing, age of sexual activity is not. Cultural stigmas and discrimination prevent unmarried women in most countries from having access to birth control, abortion, perinatal services, and social welfare programs. A vicious cycle, exacerbated by HIV, puts women into poverty and keeps them there. Since a major route of HIV transmission in women is sexual transmission, and because teenage use of contraception and STD prophylaxis is especially low, countries or communities with substantial HIV infection now observe dramatic increases in morbidity and mortality of young women. Pregnancy and HIV transmission often occur — and are prevented — through roughly the same means. Increases in either pregnancy or STDs among socially isolated teenage or young women in high-HIV-incidence areas predict later high incidence of pregnant, poorly nourished HIV infected women, whose children, regardless of serostatus, will also suffer the effects of poor nutrition.

Women's Economic Status

Women are responsible for more than half of the food production in the world, and in some areas of Africa and Asia provide up to 90 per cent of the labor involved; however, women are rarely considered as an economic force. In addition, while women constitute one third of the official labor force in the world and perform nearly two-thirds of the total official work hours, they receive only one-tenth of the world income and own less than 1 per cent of property (World Health Organization, 1985). Stereotyped cultural beliefs about the nature of 'women's work' and women's invisibility in the domestic sphere and in national statistics has resulted in development patterns that lower women's economic status while improving the status of men.

Women constitute an increasingly greater percentage of the world's poor, and female-headed households, which are increasing in number, are among the poorest of the poor, a phenomenon called the 'feminization of poverty' (World Health Organization, 1989b; Ehrenreich, Stollard and Sklar, 1982). The increased workload resulting from taking on a greater share of agricultural labor and from heading single-parent homes in both rural and urban areas without improvement in nutritional status or increased access to medical care serves to lower women's general health status even further. Women are bearing an increasing share of the burden when it comes to production of resources, but experiencing a lowering of their economic status.

The absence of women in the planning process persistently results in the takeover of once female-controlled economic activities by men; when labor-saving technologies are introduced in developing nations, men typically take over the formerly odious but now higher technology activity and relegate the women who once performed it to some other equally time-consuming and low-status activity. Consequently, women continue to perform the most grinding and unrewarding tasks and do not have access to technical skills which might be transferable, for example, in migrating from agricultural to urban areas (World Health Organization, 1985, p. 10; Pizurki *et al.*, 1987).

Finally, women's low economic status results in low participation in political life. Women often form local, grass-roots support, service, or political groups; however, these are rarely integrated even into local political structures, much less regional or national ones. There is a huge gap between Ministries of Health and grass-roots women's health activities, whether these are traditional networks or groups emerging in response to a new awareness of women's role (perhaps resulting from the activities of the Decade for Women). Only recently, and in the face of top-down programme failure and health people-power shortages, have national programs sought to cooperate with local women's groups. These new programs are often described as if the Ministries have created rather than belatedly discovered the potential of traditional women's networks.

Cultural Attitudes about Women

The cultural value of women is almost universally equated with their ability to have children, with health care and nutrition directed toward women perceived to be most likely to have children. Older women, women who choose not to have children and those who engage in professions viewed to be in conflict with the maternal role receive fewer health resources and are often actively discriminated against in ways that directly affect access to health care and information. In particular, migrant women and female sex workers experience increased difficulty in acquiring health care and increased policing through the health care system. They may face ridicule, registry, and forced sterilization or abortion.

The cultural emphasis on childbearing to the exclusion of valuing women's many other contributions to the economic, political, and social life of their community make it more difficult for women to value themselves. Women's low self-esteem and exclusion from local political and social processes are impediments to attaining higher levels of participation by women in community health and formal primary health care initiatives. Although there have been some successful programs with women's organizations in Africa, outside planners have generally had difficulty generating projects in a way that ensures female participation, except in a few programs where women were already chiefly responsible for the activity (for example, water sanitation) (Rifkin, 1990; Pizurki *et al.*, 1987). While specific, material conditions affect the health status of women, the virtually universal devaluation of women as persons is perhaps the most difficult and insidious cause of women's lower mental and physical health status.

The single most important result of the Decade for Women may have been in raising women's awareness about the importance of their role and contribution in many aspects of community, family, and social life. While many countries lack the economic means to equalize women's resources, even the richest resist improving women's status through laws and information programs targeted at social attitudes. The United States still lacks equal constitutional rights for women on the federal level and in many other countries women have only the legal standing of children or property. The nearly uniform negative valuation of women (except as child-producers) means that women lack the self-esteem, awareness, and political and social skills to effect self-help programmes envisioned by even the most sensitive planners committed to community empowerment.

On a practical level, negative attitudes toward women place them at higher risk for acquiring sexually transmitted diseases, including HIV. Universally, without regard to region, socioeconomic status, or cultural beliefs, women express an inability to obtain cooperation from their male partners in prevention measures such as condom use or shifts to non-penetrative sexual options. Women experience or fear violence, rejection by current partners, and inability to attract future partners if they demand compliance with health promotion campaigns which propose changes in sexual behavior in order to prevent contracting HIV or STDs (Branch for the Advancement of Women, 1989).

On the policy level, devaluation of women's health in general will in part determine how scarce resources are redeployed as the demands of the HIV epidemic reshape health economies. In countries experiencing recession, it is frequently the complex of social services which enable women's autonomy and health which are cut first, for example, childcare subsidies and centers or programs directed toward helping women acquire new skills to compete in the job market. Unless it is specifically targeted, women's generally lower health and mental health is unlikely to be a top priority in policy development over the next decade of economic constraint. Women's health is likely to once again be considered important only to the extent that it affects children's health or to the extent that women are needed to fill in gaps in the economy which changes in men's labor patterns have left vacant. Unless women are considered equal partners in society, they will continue to be at the bottom of the economic chain; the last to experience the 'trickle down' effects of prosperity and the first to experience 'tightening of the belt'.

Moreover, women, and especially sex workers, are erroneously viewed as the 'cause' of AIDS; too many programs are aimed either at 'controlling prostitution' or at preventing childbearing among women perceived to be at high risk. This has resulted in considerable discrimination against women who are already marginalized and stigmatized. There is little acknowledgment that women are most likely to have been infected by their boyfriends, husbands, or clients. Until women are generally seen as valuable members of society — as persons — neither national policy nor intimate interactions are likely to change.

Barriers to Women's Health

This chapter has considered the barriers to women's health common to women around the world. Denied access to many of the activities which promote a sense of self-worth, develop skills, and provide information about mental and physical health, women frequently do not even see the importance of their own well-being. Women have little or no access to HIV control or planning processes, even though they are major providers of education and primary health care in all societies. Stereotyped representations of who is 'at risk' prevent most women from realizing that they might become infected.

Gender and social roles which privilege men make it difficult for women to receive a fair share of family resources, even when they contribute most of the primary care and, in some cultures, a large percentage of the food. In particular, women have little control over sexual, reproductive, or work decisions and are subject to punishment and violence within the family. Women's lack of control over their own bodies means that they have difficulty effecting health promotion plans.

Social structures such as denial of education, exclusion from paid work, and lack of property rights prevent or inhibit women's open participation in society. Women can neither voice their concerns about issues affecting them, nor gain the skills and esteem which are part of social and political participation. Cultural and religious ideologies reinforce social roles and political structures by providing them with deeply felt rationales. Specific cultural and religious practices, especially those concerning marriage, childbearing, and sexuality, negatively affect the health of women.

International barriers, such as the under-representation of women in national Health Ministries, in organizations such as the World Health Organization, and in non-governmental organizations, mean that women have little opportunity to observe or challenge the worldwide patterns of women's health problems. Lack of prior involvement in international health efforts means that few women have the skills to analyze or suggest macro-level policy. Although women are now frequently listed as a group needing special assessment and programming, it is rarely women who effect such plans.

It was a major accomplishment for the world community to recognize that the welfare and development of all countries are dependent on the status and well-being of their women citizenry. Less well accepted is the equally important interrelation of women's social status and their health options. This complex, multi-layered connection between women's status and women's health, between women's health and the health of their families, communities, and even countries, cannot be overemphasized. Thus, while there is an immediate imperative to develop programs for counseling HIV-seropositive women, long-range programming — if it is to succeed — must also seek to empower women generally through involvement in local, national, and international HIV care and prevention initiatives. However it is precisely when the focus shifts from women's contribution to others to others' contribution to women that conflicts arise.

This chapter has presented a very general picture, highlighting the universal aspects of women's condition. The next chapter will look more closely at how one country's media represented the risk of HIV to its women. Often controlled by national interests, media representations vary considerably around the globe. However, since the US has featured so prominently in the discovery and control of HIV, the US media have been uniquely influential in creating a picture of the pandemic. The next chapter will provide a close reading of the specific cultural logic in the US media which projects certain women as risky to men or fetuses while at the same time denying the danger HIV presents to women themselves.

Chapter 5

Women at Risk[1]

'Most of the reported [cases among heterosexuals] clearly involved anal sex or intravenous drugs', [Dr. Jay A. Levy of the University of California, San Francisco] says. (*Newsweek*, 'Special Report on AIDS', 12 August 1985)

I have only normal heterosexual intercourse . . . but I've become a lot more selective about my partners. (A 'typical single woman' quoted in *People Magazine*, 'AIDS and the Single Woman', 14 March 1988)

The 30 July 1990 issue of *People* magazine featured a full cover photograph of a hopeful Ali Gertz, with the bold, black headline 'AIDS: A Woman's Story' above her head. Burned in white type over her dark sweater were the words 'Her date came with champagne, roses . . . and AIDS. Eight years later, ALI GERTZ, 24, is fighting for her life and warning women that, yes, it can happen to you. Inside: Her story and those of six other women living with the deadly disease'.

Though certainly not the first woman in her situation, Gertz, through media attention and her own decision to become publicly involved in HIV education, provided a 'real' referent for the apocryphal stories about 'average' white middle-class young women who contracted the virus through 'ordinary sexual intercourse' with men from their own class. Coming on the heels of a highly publicized New York City 'love murder' case, in which a young man of Gertz's social class killed his girlfriend during 'rough sex', the Gertz story was able to draw on a reemerging anxiety that 'nice men' harbor a variety of pathologies. The *People* magazine version of Gertz's story was able to distance itself from the tropes of films like *Fatal Attraction* because the 'new American gothic' genre — inaugurated by David Lynch's *Blue Velvet* — had shifted popular narrative attention away from the specter of a pathological female who destroys men and onto the nice-guy-gone-nuts who destroys her. *People* manages to evade the vilification of the 'promiscuous' woman common to AIDS discourse, but it succeeds only by romanticizing the spunky, well-to-do socialite who was infected with a virus of the 'Other' through a man as socially emblematic as herself. The moral is that 'ordinary' woman are not only at danger if they cross class lines, but also within the tightly guarded bounds of their own class.

The story is vague as to how Gertz's boyfriend had become infected. He seems to have had sex with men: ironically, the omnipresence of the well-groomed gay lawyer or doctor with HIV diminished the otherness of homosexuality, as long as such 'deviants' bear upper class markers. Or, *People* suggests, he might have injected designer drugs for fun. Media accounts had already established these high-tech escapes as a problem plaguing yuppies with career stress and a puritanical incapacity to pursue simpler forms of leisure. Yuppie 'use' of cocaine was less personally demeaning and socially destructive than the 'abuse' of heroin or crack which was represented as characterizing black or working-class 'street addicts' who were the real targets of America's 'war on drugs'.

Even though it reproduced many class-linked misconceptions about AIDS, the *People* version of Gertz's story fused two reportorial strategies developed during the previous seven years: sensational stories of heterosexual women's categorical vulnerability and avoidance of discussion of sexual behavior were joined dividing women into a 'general public' versus those 'at risk'. By the time of the Gertz story, women at risk were visually represented as women of color, drug injectors, or sex workers or narratively portrayed as women unable to distinguish a gay/bisexual man from a 'real' (safe) man.

By the mid 1980s, media accounts had begun to represent HIV-seropositive women of the middle class as women who had poor partner selection skills. The idea that nice girls might not be able to weed out dangerous men was crucial to the *People* version of the Gertz story. Evidence of some women's inability to sort out the good from the bad was often contained in second-hand anecdotes — interviews with friends who express suspicion about a man the protagonist had dated. Sometimes a photograph of the 'shadowy bisexual' man (or someone we are to imagine as like him) would be included with the story. Here, the reader is placed in the position of getting to meet the undiscerning woman and the man who infected her. Her judgment is indicted because the reader, having already been cued and assisted by the encoding of the heterosexual impersonator with 'gay' signifiers, can easily pick him out as 'queer'. Self-assurance allows the reader to conclude that there must be something wrong with the woman in the story if she can't tell that a man is bisexual. Playing on women's belief that 'it can't happen to me', mainstream media accounts suggest that women need only improve their skills at decoding the male body. This process of reading, with its critique of other women's readings of danger, promotes partner selection over changes in sexual repertoire as the best strategy for risk reduction.

The Risk that Could Not Speak Its Name

AIDS seemed always to be a possession of deviant groups fractured off from the mainstream, and women seemed to be the stitches holding the tattering mainstream together (mothers, wives, sisters, volunteers). Capacity to acquire HIV became a signifier of deviance: the slide from 'risk' to 'deviance' virtually disabled efforts to direct education toward women, or even recognize that women had clinical AIDS. As described in Chapter One, while there were many reported cases of women with AIDS in the first five years of the epidemic, the CDC did not count cases by gender until well after the most sensational reports on women and AIDS had appeared. These media accounts first raised the specter of pervasive infection (as in a 1985 *Life* cover which claimed, confusingly, that 'No One is Safe') and then retreated to assure the public that 'ordinary' heterosexuals were not in danger. In particular, AIDS was early said to result from anal sex itself (independent of any virus), a practice which, according to broad social perception, is 'kinky', a 'primitive form of birth control', or associated chiefly with 'prostitution'. Public discussion of heterosexuals who had contracted HIV might have broken down the homophobia and misogyny latent in the epidemiological labeling. Instead, by fusing the myth that AIDS is caused by anal sex with the myth that 'normal' heterosexuals do not engage in this practice, the category of risk/deviance expanded to include 'kinky' heterosexuals. The fundamental bifurcation, evident from the beginning of the epidemic in researchers' and the media's use of the terms 'risk groups' and 'general public', survived unchallenged because heterosexuals with AIDS were re-categorized as nominal queers.

This mystification of risk seemed to work in tandem with a reconstruction of notions of identity. Rather than remaining as a kind of silent, invulnerable norm against which the 'deviations' were constructed, the 'general public' received an identity as white, non-drug-injecting, and, especially, heterosexual. Like gay people's oppositional identity construction in relation to the homophobia of the post-war years, 'heterosexuals' seemed to form a more concrete and public identity in opposition to the claim that 'anyone can get AIDS'. This 'straight' identity sometimes worked to more clearly articulate an inchoate collective desire for 'normal intercourse' with the 'opposite sex', but as often served as a mechanism for distancing from risk of contracting the 'gay plague', and even as a position from which to advocate draconian measures against 'deviants' or to engage in hate crimes.

Once risk reduction education spelled out the specific hazards of sex, the covert but common practice of male/male sex among non-gay-identified men had somehow to be excluded from 'straight' identity. The media took an old category, 'bisexual', and revised its connotative meaning in order to account for those men who seemed incapable of taking up a stable identity and role in either the 'general [heterosexual] public' or the 'gay lifestyle'. Despite the media's new character, the indecisive bisexual, CDC epidemiology and risk reduction advice grounded in it continued to use the category 'homosexual/ bisexual male', leaving a wide interpretive space for men and women reluctant to be hailed by educational campaigns.

The notion of bisexuality evolved at least twice since the 1960s notion of 'swingers' or hippies who were essentially heterosexual men who 'chose' both male and female partners. In the post-gay-liberation era, bisexuality included women and men, but they were viewed as 'straddling the fence' until they finally 'came out' as gay or lesbian. These 'bisexuals' were partly 'in the closet' and led a 'double life', an asexual, pretend heterosexual one and a true gay/lesbian one. In the 1960s version of bisexuality, men who slept with women at all could claim the label 'straight'. In the 1970s, any sex with men marked a man as 'gay'.

Since women's sexuality is considered passive, changes in views of 'bisexuality' had little effect on the presumed 'sexual orientation' of women. The political lesbianism of 1970s feminism allowed women to claim to be 'woman-identified' even if they did not have sex with other women. In the popular mind, lesbianism seemed to have more to do with refusing to conform to gender roles than with any actual sexual behavior.

The 1960s and 1970s proposed only one masculine identity: those who failed to meet its criteria were placed in an ill defined category of otherness by default. In the 1960s, 'real men' might be allowed to dabble in sex with each other, but after the emergence of gay liberation, such activity banished them to the world of masculine pretenders. In popular discussion of HIV risk, masculinity forged an odd pact with itself. There were now two clear identities, still opposite, but based in *homogeneity* of sexual practice: straight men were those who had sex only with women and gay men were those who had sex only with men. Rather than allowing for any blurring of these boundaries, the bisexual male who emerged after Rock Hudson's much publicized death in 1985 was represented as living in a netherworld, refusing to make either of the two, now clearly marked, identifications.

If there were ever-expanding ways for men outside the core urban gay communities to *evade* identification with risk-reduction education, then women could barely have recognized themselves in the CDC accounting if they tried. If women were drug injectors their risk factor was considered a closed issue, and their sexual practices were considered redundant or irrelevant to *their* risk, though important in delineating the 'pool' of 'vessels and vectors' waiting to infect babies or men. On charts representing the breakdown of the officially counted AIDS cases by gender and risk factor, the category 'homosexual/female' was usually marked not 'zero', but 'not applicable'. Women who had sex exclusively with women were considered not at risk; 'lesbians' were widely considered to be neither drug injectors nor former or current sexual partners of men. In this same logic, 'bisexual' women were considered at risk only as the 'passive partner' during 'heterosexual intercourse' and were thus only counted as heterosexual contacts of men.

Obviously, these 'scientific' categories are deeply influenced by cultural assumptions about sexuality. Male sexuality is the only site of agency, so the bisexuality of indecision invoked in the mainstream press can only be a 'male' phenomenon. Women's sexuality is treated as totally passive. 'Heterosexual' women are understood to be partners of men rather than as agents of their own desires, and sex between women is simply considered 'not applicable' because it does not count as sex. The implicit argument is that the crucial issues of sexuality are those concerning men, a kind of patriarchal self-obsession that has still not been able to admit that, biologically speaking, women are indeed at far more risk of contracting HIV from men than vice versa.[2]

By the First International Conference on AIDS, held in Atlanta in April 1985, the association of AIDS with North American forms of deviance was under assault from another quarter. Data from African cities found that sexual intercourse between men and women was the most common risk factor among study subjects on that continent, suggesting that 'ordinary intercourse' might be an equally common modality of HIV transmission. Racist beliefs about differences in the conduct of heterosexuality were invoked to distance the North American, white heterosexual reading public from this new evidence that they might be subject to HIV infection. The cultural imperialism of Western writers prevented them from seeing the real parallels between the situation of women in 'Africa' and in Europe/America: as long as writers could blame African men it was possible to talk about the plight of women dependent on their male partners. For example, the 16 February 1987 *Time* article called 'In the Grip of the Scourge' utilizes a racist view of an 'Other' heterosexuality in order to brush away the implication that widespread infection of Western heterosexuals might be possible:

Josephine is dying because she had sexual intercourse with her late husband. A prosperous trader, he had contracted 'slim disease' . . . thousands of people in her town and the surrounding countryside have already died . . . Townspeople first attributed the mysterious disease to witchcraft. Now they know that their lovemaking is to blame.

Josephine's tragedy is the tragedy of central Africa.

Once the disease gained a foothold, it spread rapidly among Africans in the same way it has among homosexuals in the US: through sex with multiple partners.

Another key factor in the transmission of the disease is the unwillingness of many heterosexual men to change their sexual practices.

Again, men's sexuality is the concern, and women's 'plight', once mentioned, must be instantly metonymized: women's own needs and experience can never be specified or addressed.

Finally, because the original case counting considered male-to-male sex to be the primary route of transmission, men with two or more routes of exposure were represented in statistics as homosexual/bisexual. In the late 1980s, the CDC revised their categories several times to reflect cases of multiple exposure. The new categories were single-route, double-route, etc., with the basic categories remaining: male-to-male, drug injection, blood product consumption, perinatal, and partner, a category increasingly comprising women. The earliest studies demonstrated that the receptive partner in intercourse (regardless of gender) was always at much greater risk of infection. However, homophobia and sexism conspired to prevent researchers from grasping the significance of this finding: women who engage in intercourse with men are by definition 'receptive' while men who engage in intercourse with other men may be either, or both. If gay men had been considered 'partners' rather than mysterious links in a vast sex network, it might have been clear that it is their potential for bilateral transmission and not 'promiscuity' which accounts for apparent differences in rates of transmission between female and male partners of men. The clearest and most accurate ranking of probable routes of transmission would have placed needle sharers at highest risk, followed by receptive partners in intercourse, regardless of gender. Tragically, the designation of homosexual 'contact' rather than anal reception of semen ultimately mystified women's risk, analogously but inappropriately described as heterosexual 'contact', rather than vaginal or anal reception of semen.

Despite the continuing inadequacies, the new counting system made it clear for the first time that people whose sole (and therefore definitive) route of transmission was male-to-male sex only made up half of the total. If drug injection had been the privileged category in the early epidemiology (that is, if men with both 'homosexual contact' and 'drug injection' as possible exposure routes had been listed as injectors rather than homosexual), the 'homosexual' category even during the confusing first years of the epidemic would have been closer to 50 per cent of the total of cases. And, since cases among drug injectors and their female partners have continuously increased, individuals whose sole risk is male/male sex continue to decline as a percentage of total cases. Even among this number, many men do not identify with 'the gay community'; this is especially true of men of color, whose ethnic cultures have specific longstanding, if sometimes unnamed homosexual social roles.

From the mid 1980s, epidemiologists knew that an important percentage of the men infected with HIV were engaging in sex with women (half or more). Although the percentage of women among those diagnosed with AIDS was small (about 7 per cent in the mid 1980s), epidemiologists knew that about half had been infected through unprotected intercourse with male partners who had themselves been infected through needle-sharing. Given the long incubation period of HIV (set at about five years at that time)[3] and recognition that the number of infected individuals far exceeded the number of AIDS cases, this should have suggested that cases in women would dramatically increase. Nevertheless, women were rarely represented as generally at potential risk through sex, only as at risk through needle-sharing — a risk that was not only not 'sexual', but not gendered. Education aimed at drug injectors continues to emphasize needle hygiene more than condom use, and the message has been heeded: sadly, it is not unusual to find men who have stopped sharing needles but do not use condoms, or even to find needle-sharing sex partners who bleach their works but do not practice safe sex.

As described in Chapters One and Three, education was targeted at communities which public health officials believed represented individuals whose shared behaviors created a sense of group identity. For men who were willing to think of themselves as gay, promoting greater identification with their oppositional community served to increase adherence to emerging safe sex norms. This worked to some extent with drug injectors, although health officials hoped that decreases in risk taking would result in getting off drugs, returning the former user to his or her original community. But this strategy proved disastrous for women because it split AIDS education into two forms: information aimed at 'communities' described risk while information aimed at 'the general public' emphasized compassion toward people living with AIDS. Unable to easily identify with a community *as a woman* (she was de-gendered as a drug user, dangerous to others if she was a sex worker, invisible if she was in the 'general public') it became difficult for any woman realistically to consider her risk. The displacement of sex-related risk to women suggested that heterosexuality was safe by nature, requiring no modifications, not even condoms, under 'normal' circumstances.

The media further compounded women's perception of their risk through drug injection or sex in lurid stories about crack culture. Here, the 'war on drugs' joined the 'fight against AIDS', justifying additional policing of drug use without providing additional services for those who had contracted HIV. Although the media unequivocally indicted trading sex for crack as the 'cause' of skyrocketing rates of HIV infection among poor urban youth, researchers are unclear about the specific risks of HIV infection in crack culture: few crack users also inject (suggesting lower HIV risk) and the 'sex' traded seems mainly to be fellatio, generally considered to present considerably lower risk than intercourse. As suggested in Chapter Three, ethnographic studies show that women who trade sex in the crack house often also have non-crack-using, but heroin- or cocaine-injecting, partners with whom they practice intercourse. These partners are more likely to be older men who may actually be at higher risk of HIV infection than the men whose poverty leads them to smoke crack and obtain (largely oral) sex in the crack house (Ratner, 1993).

The Representation of Biology

The confusion between identity and practice was further shored up through some curious interpretations of the female body. Because the syndrome was associated with 'gay' men, and because such men were stereotyped as having only anal sex, many researchers and most popular writers initially considered women's sexual risk to be through anal sex, but not through vaginal sex. The reasoning here was tautological: if AIDS was a disease of perverted sex, than heterosexuals who got it must also be engaging in perverted sex. This association of 'heterosexual transmission' with anal sex was fallacious, a way of associating the heterosexual individuals who had acquired HIV with the paradigmatic 'homosexual' practice; 'heterosexual' — that is, penile-vaginal — intercourse is made to seem safe-by-nature by associating infected persons with some other, supposedly deviant sexual practice. The only reason offered for the hypothesized greater risk of anal intercourse was the 'rugged vagina'/ 'fragile anus' argument (see Treichler, 1988) which, while a technically accurate description, ignores the cervix as a portal of entry and rests more on bizarre folk beliefs than on any epidemiological evidence or well reasoned assessment of the biomechanics of infection. Instead of recognizing that anal sex was more common among heterosexuals than popularly believed, the 'danger of anal sex' asserted in AIDS discourse converged with the belief that 'nice girls don't' to produce a fatal bit of folklore among heterosexuals that vaginal intercourse carried no risk.

The disappearance of women into imprecise or politically charged categories like 'heterosexual', 'partners of', or even 'prostitute' and 'IVDU' only reflected on the level of representation what was occurring at the level of research and clinical practice. Women are diagnosed later in their disease process because they generally receive less health care and receive it later than male counterparts and because many physicians still have difficulty imagining that a woman they are treating might be presenting HIV-related symptoms. Doctors' misperceptions are redoubled because a range of seriously disabling or fatal gynecological sequelae to HIV infection were not counted as 'symptoms' in the CDC's definitional hierarchy until 1993. Unlike night sweats or weight loss, once non-definitive, but now red flags for HIV infection, persistent vaginal infections did not lead most clinicians down the path to a diagnosis of HIV infection.

What Women Need

Women's concerns have been erased from AIDS policy and media accounts because women are not considered to be persons. Women, and especially women's bodies, are decontextualized from women's concrete social existence, and treated as of concern only insofar as they affect men or children. To put it bluntly, women are either vaginas or uteruses, and curiously, never both at the same time. It is as if there were a great sea of undifferentiated (but generically male) bodies which, at particular moments — 'sex' (always recreational) — or for a particular purpose — procreation (never to involve pleasure) — suddenly take on two different genders. The women who emerged in the context of sex were considered 'prostitutes' or 'loose women', and the ones who become childbearers seem never to engage in 'sex'.

A 12 August 1985 *Newsweek* article illustrates dramatically this split: the left page features a large but fuzzy night shot of 'prostitutes' 'working the streets in New York: Some experts fear that prostitutes might turn out to be carriers who could further fuel the epidemic'. On the facing page are smaller photographs of pubescent Ryan White and baby Matthew Kozup, who both contracted HIV through blood products. Lest the reader fail to make the connection between sex and blood donation (weak at best), or even assume that these boys' mothers were sex workers, the article continues: 'Any future argument for unrestrained sexual life will have to take into account that it has dire new consequences — not only for those adults who freely choose it but for children like Ryan White'. 'Prostitutes' are problematic only as sex partners, not as childbearers: the writer seems never to have considered that sex workers are mothers, too. After all, sex work is a reasonably well-paying way to support their children and be home during the day. The writer could have suggested that sex workers' children are at risk from infected johns, but this would only have located the source of infection in the one place mainstream society cannot believe it exists: the willful refusal to wear condoms on the part of 'ordinary' US men.

Media and public health concern for childbearers is less with the welfare of the woman than with that of her unborn child. A 23 September 1985 *Newsweek* article, 'The AIDS

Conflict', goes so far as to construct an epidemiological category (mother with AIDS) that has never appeared in CDC counts: 'Most of the cases [among children] represent children who were born to a *mother with AIDS*, a category that seems likely to grow with the spread of the disease among intravenous drug users' (emphasis added). A 27 April 1987 *Time* article summarizing the CDC's first published report on women and AIDS (which had appeared in the *Journal of the American Medical Association* the previous week; *Time* appears to have rewritten a press release for its first major article on women and AIDS) also lays bare the assumptions about the real issues to be addressed in women's risk for HIV:

> Though women account for less than 7% of all US AIDS victims, their cases have a special significance . . . By studying these cases, researchers can get clues about how rapidly the disease is spreading among heterosexuals and among children, most of whom contract AIDS from infected mothers . . . No less striking was the study's finding that more than 70% of AIDS cases in women occurred among blacks and Hispanics. Indeed, a woman who is black is 13 times as likely as one who is white to fall victim, and 90% of infants born with AIDS are black or Hispanic.

As if this did not condemn women enough, the *Time* article cites an editorial accompanying the *JAMA* report as claiming that 'The potential future danger of AIDS is less compelling [to poor, minority women] than the day to day problems of poverty and drug use'. It seemed impossible to acknowledge that women themselves might need help.

The Always Already Infected

How either the vagina-body or the uterus-body became infected in the first place was never addressed: readers were left with the impression that particular, isolated women were somehow always already infected. The reality that it is mostly men — clients, husbands, boyfriends, needle-sharing partners — who infect women was ignored. When men are mentioned as a danger it is through the invocation of the (exceptional) bisexual man, or as a reminder that a woman (who will, of course, be 'promiscuous') will have to figure out some way to deal with getting him to use a condom. Conversely, advice to men about using condoms centers almost exclusively on the risk to them of sex for payment.

Risk reduction advice reveals its complicity in attitudes about sexuality that disadvantage women. Lists of risk factors in educational material aimed at heterosexuals include 'having sex with a prostitute', while having sex with 'johns' is absent. There is no admonition for men to protect sex workers by using condoms, only dire warnings about the danger of being infected in such a commercial transaction. Certainly, community-based organizers and educators emphasize the importance of condom use as a protection for sex workers. However, there is a slightly bizarre logic behind asking prostitutes to risk their income by getting men to use condoms, especially since public health officials seem to believe that condoms serve to protect the men. This amounts to a tax on sex workers, or perhaps a rebate to the male client, who, for the sake of the epidemic, must purchase supposedly 'inferior' experiences of sex: intercourse or oral sex while wearing a condom. The implication, and indeed the practice, of public health is to disregard the safety of women sex workers because they are viewed only as sexual receptacles, presumed to be already infected.

When women are not vaginas waiting to infect men, they are uteruses, waiting to infect fetuses. The obsessive concern with preventing conception by HIV-positive women, or by any woman who might be perceived to be at risk of contracting HIV, is often first invoked through the specter of millions of infected babies. Most media reports start by citing statistics predicting huge numbers of infected babies, numbers which usually confuse studies in which newborns are tested to indirectly discover HIV seroprevalence rates in women with studies of the number of truly infected infants. Because it is easier to obtain permission to test newborns than their adult mothers, most estimates of seroprevalence of women giving birth derive from findings from the unlinked testing of their babies. Accurate testing of the serostatus of the infants themselves can occur only later, since it takes about eighteen months before the infant has her/his own immune system.

Once the reader is horrified by the prospect of an 'AIDS generation', as one poster purporting to represent infected infants calls it, a curious tautology is proposed. Without ever suggesting that an HIV seropositive woman might rationally calculate the risks of pregnancy, and failing to recognize that most women did not discover their serostatus until late in a prenatal care process, the media suggest that by virtue of having been wanton enough to contract HIV, a seropositive woman is incapable of making an informed and reasonable pregnancy choice. The fact that an HIV-seropositive woman chooses to start or continue a pregnancy is taken as evidence of her immorality. In fact couples in which one or both partners are HIV-seropositive might view the risk of childbearing as a fair one to take. The best recent studies suggest that there is a 20 to 60 per cent chance of the child being infected. Exact figures are complicated because the women studied were at different stages of HIV infection during their pregnancies. Few studies have controlled for stage of infection, and most studies are of small cohorts. A French study (Boue *et al.*, 1990), which showed an overall 33 per cent transmission rate, grouped mothers by clinical features of their HIV infection (CD4 count, positive p24 antigenemia, and high replication rate of HIV in culture) to determine whether stage of infection affected perinatal transmission. Women with features suggestive of low infectivity gave birth to infected infants (determined by follow-up fifteen months later) in about 20 per cent of cases. Women with features suggestive of high infectivity gave birth to infected infants in about 60 per cent of cases.

But worse, when the issue of childbearing decisions by discordant couples (man HIV-seropositive, woman HIV-seronegative) is raised in documents like the World Health Organization's 1991 HIV counseling guidelines (aimed principally at developing nations who are the agency's main clients), the main counseling issue is identified as preventing the infection of the child. The reality that the seronegative woman will also become infected in the process of conception (i.e., during 'sex') is ignored.

The WHO guidelines and similar recent advice chose to ignore the wealth of evidence showing that HIV seropositive women will continue to choose to bear children and for a variety of reasons which counseling will largely not affect. This pattern was clearly established by the 1989 Fifth International

Conference on AIDS (Montreal) where numerous studies described a consistent pattern of decisions to pursue pregnancy among infected women who participated in a variety of counseling programs.[4] Faced with a 40 to 80 per cent chance of bearing a *non-infected* child, these do not seem like such irrational or immoral decisions.

Finally, research on drug injection and advice to injectors also ignores the gendered power relations among needle-sharers. Although there is little data on needle-sharing risk by gender, research on drug injection in general suggests that men predominate in this form of drug use. In a study of methadone clinics on which I served as ethnographer, it appeared that male injectors (except those whose long term relationships are with women they inject with) preferred not to form sexual relationships with female injectors, an existing subcultural prejudice exacerbated by the 'choose carefully' (as opposed to 'clean your works') educational message which linked *sexual* risk with particular kinds of people. In addition, women injectors said that their male partners insisted on injecting them, and were reluctant to explain how to obtain and prepare drugs and injection apparatus. Women had to covertly learn how to 'hit' themselves instead of availing themselves of the apprenticeship system available to men. Women saw their exclusion from full participation in the larger drug culture as men's way of maintaining power over their female partners; women who share predominantly with men are engaged in a gendered power relationship which disadvantages women.

When 'People' Doesn't Fit

Women's needs are also elided because they are viewed only as exceptions or variations to generalities about 'people living with AIDS', a term which always implicitly refers to men. We don't for example, say 'men living with AIDS', or even 'men and women living with AIDS', but 'people living with AIDS', and when necessary specify 'women living with AIDS'. The concerns and issues of people living with AIDS orient toward men's social situation, men's bodies, and men's needs. Women are thought to have 'special needs' when the basic male-oriented model is shown to be clearly incapable of accounting for their presence or experience. This is in no way to undervalue the importance of the People Living With AIDS (PLWA) movement, its conscious attempts to involve women, and its concrete role in improving the lives of women. But the movement would have been different if it had risen out of women's experience of the epidemic.

For example, in order to reject the label of 'victim', the PLWA movement helps individuals frame a new identity combining the 'coming out' model commonly understood in gay culture with the method of 'telling your story' developed in Alcoholics Anonymous and Narcotics Anonymous culture, both of which empower the individual by helping them to reframe an identity which society labels as bad or immoral. To the extent that individuals can relate to this model, the PLWA movement is empowering. However, women, especially those infected through 'ordinary' intercourse with their husband or boyfriend, have difficulty claiming this new identity; although women's reproductive capacities have sometimes been viewed as sources of increased fragility, women as a class are not labelled deviant or sick as are homosexuals and drug injectors. The conditions of poverty and isolation which many men experience *because* of their AIDS diagnosis were already the lived experience of poor women. For women, an AIDS diagnosis usually does not cause the change in social standing or identity that it does for self-identified gay men.

This individual empowerment model has become the trend in most Western counseling and service delivery agencies. The model assumes that the major problem of the person living with AIDS is making the behavior and attitude changes which 'safe sex', 'recovery', and the patient role require, and assumes that the best way of supporting the person living with AIDS is to provide help from paraprofessionals and volunteer befrienders. While paraprofessionals and befrienders augment a system of supports for men, they may disempower a woman or her support networks by introducing someone with a perceived higher social status and connections to formal public health surveillance systems, especially if the paraprofessionals and befrienders are men. This gender-biased model may serve to make a woman's situation worse by encouraging separation from her existing family system and informal women's networks.

Why We Can't Talk About Prevention

Perhaps the most deadly erasure of women's needs has been in the area of HIV infection prevention. Certainly, the tendency to view women as either vaginas or uteruses enables educators and policymakers to avoid the issue of how and why women are infected in the first place. It is hard not to see the workings of an adolescent male sexual psychology in this desire to avoid the idea that sex can lead to conception and, at the same time, to refuse to ask where babies come from. Sex is implicitly reconstituted as a man's right and a woman's obligation, with women responsible both for protecting men from disease and for avoiding the consequences of transmission to a man's child. From the 'active', male perspective, risk is equated with women, not with particular heterosexual practices. From the woman's perspective, a husband or boyfriend may be at risk from someone else (a needle-sharing partner, a 'homosexual' partner, or a 'vagina'), and her child might be at risk from her ('uterus'), but the twist in the logic of safe sex which encourages heterosexuals to view unpaid intercourse as 'safe' makes it difficult for a woman to perceive *herself* as at risk.

As discussed above, women's knowledge of serostatus *often precedes* their realization that they might be at risk because women generally discover their serostatus during antenatal care or after a male partner is diagnosed with an HIV-related illness. The positive community concern and support for testing among gay men which enables identification of risk, considered decisions about testing, and follow-up medical intervention do not exist for most women. Women simply discover, almost by accident, that they have been infected. This is no coincidence, since the media and counseling programs describe women as either at risk through socially-disapproved-of 'dangerous' sex and drug use, or as apparently always and already infected. This construction of dangerous sex prevents most women from perceiving themselves to be at risk of HIV infection because when they are having sex with men they 'love', they view themselves as engaging in 'ordinary' or 'normal', and therefore 'safe', heterosexual intercourse.

A Queer Sort of Resistance

Ironically, the initial societal construction of AIDS as a disease of dangerous sexuality in part *enabled* gay men to identify the mechanisms of change: changing to 'safe sex' behaviors constituted a new, politically resistive space of identity for many gay men. Having already proudly claimed 'pride' in what society viewed as a perversion, it was not that hard defiantly to claim pride in a new 'safer' sexuality now that society had used AIDS to condemn homosexuality once again. As a gay man in a Boston-based organizing project called 'Safe Company' said to me:

> Every time I have safe sex, I feel like I'm getting back at straight society. I have a lot of sex, and I feel like I'm avenging the deaths of my friends. It's like I can say see, I can still be queer and you can't make me die.

I don't want to idealize gay male culture, nor underplay the trauma many gay men have experienced as they watch friends and lovers get sick, and as they grapple with the very complex and often painful process of re-establishing identity on the other side of 'safe sex'. But it is important to understand, on the ideological level, why gay men and gay communities can still fight back, in order to understand the depth of resistance to change among members of the 'general public', a resistance to change that is far more hazardous to women than to men. Why, at the very core of heterosexual identity, is there an incapacity to understand what is being said about safe sex? It seems baffling that a relatively small change — use of a condom or, at most, shifting to non-intercourse forms of sexual pleasure — should be greeted, especially by heterosexual men, as if it were tantamount to castration. The media, probably the major source of information for those outside the 'risk groups' who have received targeted or community-generated education, construct homosexual personhood, homosexual activities of any sort, even homosexual 'safe sex', as at least partially risky; but they depict only particular *heterosexual individuals* as risky, and acts of 'ordinary' heterosexual intercourse as never risky. While the logic promoted within gay male culture views particular acts as risky and to be modified or avoided, the logic within heterosexual culture remains one that views certain individuals as risky and to be avoided. Within gay male culture, there has been a massive effort to reinvent homosexuality and homosexual identity as 'safe sex' while retaining longstanding gay culture values, including the acceptance of promiscuity and experimental sex. The lapel badge which reads 'safe sex slut' is not viewed as contradictory within gay male culture.

This effort to ideologically reconstruct gay sex as safe sex seems to have partially succeeded; and for heterosexuals, too, 'safe sex' is now interpreted by many as applying largely to 'kinky', that is 'gay', 'bisexual', or 'promiscuous' sex. By sharp contrast, heterosexuals seem to have gone to great lengths to deny a place for safe sex within heterosexual identity. The very sexual techniques which make 'queer' sex safe seem to ruin heterosexual sex: 'real sex' is that which does not require any of the techniques or latex accoutrements of 'safe sex'. There is a dichotomy between 'normal' heterosexual sex and 'safe sex', at least conceptually.

Heterosexuals routinely invoke HIV antibody testing as a mechanism to determine when to use a condom and this misperception of testing, promoted by the media and public health system alike, is tragic and fatal for women. In addition, heterosexuals who initially use condoms with a partner seem to abandon them when a 'relationship' (however defined) is established. Studies suggest that there are important disparities between heterosexuals' willingness to use condoms with new or 'suspect' partners and their willingness to use them in primary or long-term relationships. Ironically, *ceasing to use condoms* may signal trust and commitment for heterosexuals (Gallois *et al.*, 1990). There is some evidence that this is becoming true among some gay men as well (Stall *et al.*, 1990), a phenomenon I have elsewhere described as the 'heterosexualization of gay sex'.[5]

Of course, criticism of heterosexual ideology is not new: feminists have long made similar claims about how it prevents women from controlling their bodies and lives. But this is not a call to abandon cross-gender sexual relations. The typical rebuttal to criticism of heterosexual relations, and especially heterosexual intercourse, is that if men and women stopped 'doing it' the human race would become extinct. The far right has capitalized on just this argument, but with an interesting twist. Gene Antonio, author of an early and widely distributed right-wing book on AIDS, argues that homosexuals should be quarantined because 'safe sex' is a plot not only to allow homosexuals to 'continue their filthy practices' but to cause 'self-extinction of mankind' (Antonio, 1986, p. 148). To counter arguments that he might be homophobic, Antonio argues that gay people and the CDC (mysteriously controlled by the 'homosexual lobby') are *hetero*phobic: by promoting safe sex for everyone they are creating dissent between men and women and aversion toward heterosexual intercourse. This seems paranoid and silly, but only displays in relief a much more pervasive but less articulated fear which undercuts the efficacy of risk-reduction education.

Pop sexology gurus Masters, Johnson, and Kolodny (1988) pulled out all the stops, suggesting that the fundamental difference between gay sexuality and heterosexuality lies not in the gender of object choice, but in attitudes toward the meaning of safe sex. Instead of safe sex being a form of liberation from fears of infection, a practice of pleasure, the authors present safe sex as something to be dreaded, something which turns sex into a confrontation with danger. It turns out that safe sex equals queer sex, and the fear of perversion is transformed into a fear of safe sex. This homophobic calculus allows Masters and Johnson to conclude with a bizarre formulation that opposes *safe* and *natural* sex. They are particularly disgusted by the technical implications of safe sex, and never even consider the non-intercourse practices of safe sex as potentially satisfying elements in the heterosexual repertoire. The following quotation from their book reveals most dramatically this deep-seated fear of the *cultural* danger of safe sex:

> Sex partners of uncertain [HIV antibody] testing status could . . . wear disposable plastic gloves during all intimate moments. These gloves, after all, aren't too different from condoms. Yet we are unwilling to seriously entertain such an outlandish notion — right now, it seems so unnatural and artificial as to violate the essential dignity of humanity. (Masters *et al.*, 1988, p. 118)

This is strong language to use about a little latex. It is doubly ironic given that Masters and Johnson have long preached the malleability of human sexual behavior. Why is a latex glove any more unnatural or undignified than performing daily exercises to tighten vaginal muscles, or step-by-step exercises to help delay ejaculation? Masters and Johnson propose that heterosexuals do any act they choose, as long as they have had three (yes, specifically three) negative HIV antibody tests, spaced three months apart. Of course, they note, heterosexuals must abstain from sexual intercourse during this time in order for the test results to be valid. For Masters and Johnson, safe sex is a punishment for those who 'fail' or refuse to take the test, or who can't abstain for the nine months which they view as sufficient to eliminate the possibility of test errors. This not-too-subtly redraws the line between a homosexuality which they once studied and deemed normal, and a heterosexuality which they now want to preserve as natural. Even condoms are unacceptable, not only because they are not '100% safe' but because 'many couples find the postorgasmic glow a time of tenderness in which they want to lie quietly together with their genitals still in union, they run a distinct risk of having just such spillage [of the semen from around the now 'receded' penis] occur' (Masters *et al.*, 1988, p. 116).

On one side, the authors lovingly describe participants in a 'natural' heterosexuality which has no limits, but can accept no latex. On the other side are all those people who, because they are truly queer or merely nominally queer, are condemned to safe sex, that latex-ridden set of activities which dehumanizes its practitioners. This barely concealed homophobia sweeps even aberrant heterosexuals under the banner of perversion, and naturalizes the condomless heterosexual intercourse which women need to be challenging. The authors use precisely the terms which have always been used to describe both non-conformist women and homosexual sex: dehumanized, unnatural, artificial, not to be taken seriously.

The reified heterosexuality invoked here is widely recognizable either as the beacon by which to gauge inadequacies, or the monument to defy. As an ideological system and set of symbolically overdetermined practices, heterosexuality is not new, but it is newly dangerous for women. Women's efforts to wrest control over their bodies by fighting *for* legalized birth control and abortion, organizing *against* sexual violence and sexual harassment, and working to achieve women's agency and freedom to seek sexual pleasure, are in jeopardy because the logic of safe sex under the sign of AIDS has once again constituted heteromasculinity as exempt from change. The terror at the heart of men's unwillingness to wear a condom is equalled only by the power heterosexual men have to make someone else — usually a woman — protect them from themselves. But while the men who have fallen victim to that trap called heterosexual masculinity may deserve sympathy, the fact is that while men fear for their sexual identity, their women partners need to fear contracting HIV. It is easy to find fault with men who lie about their past to their wives and girlfriends, but it is not just a few unredeemed men who are the problem. At fault is the continuing construction of heterosexuality and specifically heterosexual intercourse as 'safe by nature' which prevents women from protecting themselves. Until heterosexuality means more than intercourse, and can always accommodate a condom, women will be forced to make case-by-case, situational demands on men. The paradox is this: heterosexual intercourse can only be truly 'safe' when its male practitioners are just *queer enough* to wear a condom.

This chapter has explored the US media construction of women's HIV risk. The final chapter returns to the problem of creating meaningful programs for women in this and other ideological contexts.

Notes

1 An earlier version of this chapter appeared in Squire (1993).
2 A review (Alexander *et al.*, 1990) of studies of 'heterosexual' transmission, i.e., male-to-female or female-to-male transmission, noted that while data from developing countries (largely Africa) and US/Europe differ, the latter showed higher rates of male-to-female than female-to-male transmission. The nine studies of female-to-male transmission had samples of less than thirty, while the thirteen studies of male-to-female transmission had samples ranging from 56 to 164. Epidemiological reviews at the end of 1988 showed that in the US, male-to-female transmission accounted for some 2 per cent of all AIDS cases, while female-to-male cases represented 0.6 per cent (1,757 versus 539 cases). Thus, examining epidemiological counts of cases reported by gender and by route of transmission, and biological factors such as alterations in vaginal chemistry during the menstrual cycle and response to decreasing function of the immune system, women are considered more consistently infectable than infectious.
3 The theorized length of incubation increased as researchers were able to monitor over longer periods of time. Researchers currently set time from infection to first symptoms among Westerners who have received adequate health care at twelve years.
4 Sunderland *et al.* (1989) found that 'HIV infection does not have a clear impact, if any, on reproductive decisions in this population [New York City low-income women]. Psychosocial and economic variables may have a greater influence' and

Wiznia *et al.* (1989) had similar findings among low-income women in the Bronx: 'Neither the presence of an HIV infected older child nor HIV associated symptoms in HIV infected pregnant women appear to influence decision making concerning termination of pregnancy'. Anderson *et al.* (1989) found that 'Knowledge of HIV infection was not associated with pregnancy termination or prevention of subsequent pregnancy'; Kaplan *et al.* (1989) found that, especially among women who were infected with HIV during sex with men, 'pregnancy continues to occur frequently' despite repeated counseling about 'safe sex'; and Schneck *et al.* (1989) found that 'Despite counseling for risks associated with HIV, a high percent of HIV seropositive women in this cohort became pregnant an average of 8 mo. after delivering an HIV seropositive child'. Research in Zaire proved no different. Hassig *et al.* (1989) found that '71% wanted more children . . . (mean desired family size = 5.2)' and urged that 'counselling services for HIV seropositive women in Kinshasa must be prepared to address the current low level of contraceptive usage and the definite pro-natalist sentiment in the population reflected by the high levels of desired and completed fertility'.

5   Many straight people and some gay men find it hard to imagine that there are many gay men who never or rarely engage in anal sex, since that practice has become over-associated with gay men, at least in the 1970s and 1980s. I have attempted to trace recent changes among gay men about what constitutes 'real gay sex,' and argued that these shifts may be related to educational and media representations of the epidemic. In brief, I argue that increased discourse within gay male culture about condom use overemphasized the centrality of intercourse, replacing a late 1970s view of gay sex as a veritable menu of possible delights only one of which was 'butt fucking' with a hierarchy of acts assembled through varying interpretations of risk which simultaneously vilified anal intercourse and suggested it was the 'ultimate' gay-identity-bestowing act. This shift, along with admonitions to form monogamous pair bonds, attempted to bring gay sexual identity in line with that in the dominant culture, apart from the gender of the object choice. This 'heterosexualizing' of gay identity was schizophrenic: it shifted the focus away from 'safe practices' which had been widely accepted in gay culture ('mutual masturbation', fantasy play) and which heterosexuals largely still view as impractical 'substitutes' for intercourse; and it demanded that gay men focus more on the sexual act alleged to be most dangerous, and pair bond in a society in which same-sex marriage is not sanctioned. It may also be that increased visibility of the diverse gay practices has made it more possible for heterosexuals to imagine a wider range of pleasures (Patton, 1990).

Chapter 6

Planning for Women

Planners, program developers, and activists encounter several paradoxes when they begin to formalize and conceptualize women's role and needs in order to frame appropriate responses to the HIV pandemic. Some advocate for programs which address women as a special group, usually for the purposes of education and improving risk reduction strategies. Others seek removal of gender-based barriers to treatment or care, for example, lifting the exclusion of women from AIDS treatment drug trials, or including as diagnostic the range of gynecological complications of HIV, as recently occurred in the US. On one hand, women can benefit from claiming status as a special group, but on the other, designating women as a special group can fuel negative stereotypes and increase discrimination. Policymakers feel frustrated when special programs created for women are greeted with accusations of discrimination, or when 'gender-blind' programs are seen as insensitive by women who use or need information or services. Women's dual social status as childbearers and as persons further complicates program and policy design. Women's specific needs in relation to childbearing (which are perceived to be largely biomedical, but are also significantly social and cultural) are too often turned around to exclude women from other programs or social roles (for example, many societies do not recognize women's desire for and right to education unrelated to their childbearing role).

As detailed in Chapter Three, the paradoxes are even more evident in programs for and policies regarding sex work. On one hand, women sex workers could be understood as constituting a work-related community with its own cultural values. Seen in this way, as they are by many sex workers and their advocates, sex-work-related projects present an important opportunity to influence the behavior of two groups: sex workers and their clients. However, cultural stereotypes which suppose that sex workers are different than 'other women' make it difficult for many policymakers and planners to imagine programs which transfer the knowledge sex workers have gained to their female peers who are not employed in sex work.

Because HIV/AIDS is widely perceived as stemming from perverse or abnormal sexual behavior (see Chapter Five), few women identify themselves as at risk in the course of their 'ordinary' relationships; they view themselves as practicing 'normal' sex with their male partners and have difficulty believing that these partners may have engaged in risk behaviors. Outside gay male culture and the community of sex workers, groups who recognize the need to modify sexual behaviors to reflect changing norms and knowledge, most heterosexuals can think of no reason to reorganize their sexual behavior in order to avoid risk.

The implicit message in safe sex campaigns and in research (which focuses chiefly on female sex workers' potential for transmitting HIV rather than their much greater risk of acquiring it from male partners) is that risk reduction is about preventing men from acquiring HIV and preventing women from passing HIV to a child. Until condom use is considered the norm, rather than a punitive reaction to perceived deviancy, and until sexual expression can 'naturally' take forms other than intercourse, women are unlikely to be able to change their practices until after they discover they are HIV-seropositive. The crucial link, preventing women from acquiring HIV in the first place, is only haphazardly addressed.

As suggested in Chapter Three, a major difficulty with adapting counseling and education programs from gay male communities is that women do not, for the most part, exist in intentionally constructed, socially identifiable subcultures defined by gender: from the standpoint of society, women are supposed to exist in a family unit, dispersed among the men and children with whom they share reciprocal responsibility. In some cultures, and increasingly, there are socially sanctioned women's organizations which enable women to create norms and beliefs about their roles and relationships. However, unlike gay men, who can expect to interact with other men who have similar values and who have received similar forms of education and counseling, women encounter as sexual and procreative partners men who have received no counseling or education comparable to theirs. In so far as behavioral and gender-role changes are required, women must not only work through their own concerns and challenge their own beliefs, but also confront the men they relate to with virtually no support either from those men or from other women. Women who have sex with women face additional social stigma and their needs are rarely recognized in educational campaigns.

Thus, for the purposes of education and risk-reduction promotion women should be conceptualized as living in two or more normative communities. Depending on the organization of sexuality (how compulsory is heterosexuality? how much non-sexual interaction occurs between men and women? how much mutual understanding and support do women give each other?) women's beliefs and norms about sex will derive in part from a group comprised of women peers and in part from their interactions with men.

Even for women whose sexuality is largely organized in relation to women, the concepts and norms they perceive stemming from 'heterosexual' culture will play a strong role in their sense of norms outside that culture. They may adopt, reject, or modify perceived 'heterosexual' norms in addition to forming social patterns and behavioral norms that have little to do with expectations of the perceived 'heterosexual' culture. Practically speaking, women who view themselves as lesbians or as bisexual may prefer to process the shifting sexual norms surrounding HIV prevention in groups comprised of other lesbian or bisexual women. Chapter Three considered the ways in which lesbian women have understood their relation to risk reduction, as well as tracing the epidemiological confusion over sex between women and lesbians' and bisexual women's identities.

Drug using networks, sex-work related networks, community of origin and community of residence, should also be considered as potential additional sites of differing norms. Bridging the gap between the various places where a woman may forge sexual and relational bonds is the greatest challenge to HIV counseling and risk-reduction programs: like the migrants whose movement between normatively different situations is dramatic, a woman's determination to effect risk reduc-

tion in one arena in her life where she forms relationships —
especially if that is stereotyped as a 'dangerous' place — may not
lead to effecting a risk reduction strategy that is successful in all
the places where she may form relationships. There will be
inherent contradictions and conflicts between different efforts
aimed at shifting sexual and drug use mores: while woman-
centered programs tend to improve women's self-esteem and
their desire to make risk-reducing changes, these wishes are often
met with confusion or hostility by male partners. Family or
couple-centered programs coordinate the partners' mutual
wishes to reduce risk, but often leave unchallenged the status
differentials which have placed women at a disadvantage to
begin with (Cohen and Wiseberg, 1990).

Existing Initiatives

The major global initiative dealing with women to date has
been the work of the World Health Organization's Global
Programme on AIDS (GPA) with prostitutes. This work
recognizes that sex workers, and especially women sex workers,
have been blamed for the epidemic in many parts of the world.
Some of the most impressive programs for women have occurred
among sex workers who serve as educators and counselors and
who support each other in the shift toward demanding risk
reduction and especially condom use with clients. In some
settings, such programs have begun to include formal education
of male clients, some of whom have also become involved in
education and self-education. Most female sex workers are also
wives/partners and mothers, and thus face the same relationship
and childbrearing decisions as women who are not sex workers.
The stigma attached to sex work has overshadowed the level of
risk to *all* women through 'ordinary intercourse' with the men
they know best: boyfriends and husbands. The perceived separ-
ateness of communities of sex workers has prevented transferring
their excellent work to projects for and by women generally. In
the face of these WHO-GPA initiatives, some governments in
Europe and Africa have begun to change their policies in
relation to 'prostitution' and improve programs to help sex
workers. But the motives for the increase in programs for sex

workers are mixed: too often, the unspoken message is that sex workers are responsible for the dispersion of HIV into 'mainstream' society.

Programs aimed at improving maternal and child health and increasing family planning are the second major form of HIV programming for women. While adding HIV education components to existing training and advocacy projects is important, expanding existing programs will largely reach women who may have already been infected, will affect only the classes and groups of women who already seek prenatal or child health care, and will increase agency mediation of education. While this approach will aid many women, local branches of maternal and child health and family planning programs should assess the specific, immediate aspects of women's lives which enable or disable risk reduction decisions. Agencies should be aware that their counseling style may not be adequately geared toward enhancing traditional coping systems which women will need in order to obtain information and primary care through informal routes: maternity-related and family planning programs have not been designed to deal with the wide ranging stresses and community crises which are part of the HIV pandemic.

Few protocols for counseling people with HIV contain specific information about, or analysis of, women's special problems: in general, they reduce women's issues to childbearing decisions rather than self-protection from HIV infection. Formal counseling for women must take into account that women generally make less use of medical systems than do men, especially services other than perinatal care, and are less able to follow through on health care procedures. Data from the US HIV testing centers show that women are very unlikely to return for their second appointment, when they would receive their test result and develop a risk reduction plan. Apparently, programs are not sufficiently accessible or women experience discomfort with the testing process (Nelson *et al.*, 1990; Norris *et al.*, 1990)

A third major international effort concerns integrating the work of non-governmental organizations with that of national governments, pressing both to include women and those familiar with women's needs in their planning. GPA's first meeting and conference on NGO involvement in AIDS work (March 1989) included women working in general AIDS projects and women involved in programs specifically for women. An outcome of this conference was the initiation of a small grants programme (since discontinued), an excellent opportunity for supporting and assessing small, local programming for and by women. However, it has proved difficult to link small women's groups with the larger NGOs, which have traditionally overlooked women's needs.

A subsequent consultation between GPA and women-oriented NGOs (December 1989) produced consensus that NGOs, governments, and GPA must recognize that most grass-roots efforts by women are not affiliated with any larger groups, and are often not even associated with the women-oriented NGOs. Viable projects are often invisible outside their locales, difficult to find by groups willing to fund small projects, and difficult to duplicate in other places. Some of the most effective local projects, which could be evaluated and modified for implementation in other places, do not perceive themselves to have the status of 'program' and certainly do not understand themselves to be non-governmental organizations which might be eligible for grant support. Funding agencies have been reluctant to give money to groups with no formal ties to larger groups and no clear track record, and evaluation techniques are biased toward traditionally organized projects. Governments and funding agencies must remove this kind of institutional barrier to women's participation which results from local projects' lack of recognizable formal structure. They must be willing to develop unorthodox relationships with successful, autonomous small projects, and must employ and accept non-traditional means for evaluating and expanding them.

Government health education divisions have also begun to incorporate women and women's issues into HIV educational materials and programs. Innovative programs for and by women have been lauded at recent international conferences on HIV and AIDS education. However, most government research and evaluation continues to focus on large-scale, quantitative assessment of knowledge, attitudes, beliefs, and practices (KABPs), which cannot assess the role or potential of existing community infrastructures and programs. The reality that many women have information and 'intentions' to practice risk-reducing behaviors, but are unable to effect change, is well-documented. Less clear is why and how women do manage to make changes, a phenomenon which must be studied qualitatively in specific local contexts. In addition, while there is broad recognition that women play a critical role in providing informal health education in all societies, their knowledge and expertise has been under-utilized: excessively professionalized programs, especially counseling programs which replace local, trusted sources of information with external paraprofessionals, eliminate women's mechanisms for obtaining sensitive support, and erode their social power.

Information and programs from nursing services and agencies have been more cognizant of the reality that it is women who provide the bulk of informal primary health care. Although there is fairly good documentation of informal networks in countries with less extensive and lower-technology professional health services, little is known about women's networks in settings where medicine is highly professionalized and high-technology-oriented. Developed and developing countries could both benefit from supporting and enhancing informal mutual self-care and support systems for women with HIV. These networks could also form the core of counseling efforts concerning childbearing, sexuality, and treatment options, using existing modes of information exchange and decisionmaking systems rather than replacing them with professionals who may lack knowledge of a locale or be excluded from its processes.

Many existing policies mention but do not fully evaluate and incorporate women's differing needs. For example, blood screening technical norms fail to recognize gender and regional differences in who receives blood products, in particular failing to account for the high association between women's anemia and transfusion in developing countries. Given the unlikelihood of wide implementation of effective screening, transfusion as the primary treatment for anemia and malnutrition should be reconsidered. While this is obviously a long-term project and one requiring considerable research and intersectorial planning, it is essential to begin now to address the cyclical effects that HIV-exacerbated malnutrition will have, especially in parts of the world where women are the primary food producers, but also the primary recipients of blood products. Malnourished women will seek medical care, possibly become HIV-infected as a result of treatment, thereby become less able to manage subsistence agriculture responsiblities, and become increasingly reliant on other women in their extended family networks. Given that it continues to be extremely difficult for rural women in developing countries to enter into the formal economies, their collective economic and social status will continue to fall. Thus, the subtle gender differences that link nutrition, subsistence agriculture, and blood transfusion may dramatically affect rural women in developing countries.

In addition, HIV screening and contact tracing guidelines advocate cultural sensitivity without recognizing the ways in which such programs, in their design or implementation, may actively discriminate against women or may be denied or irrelevant to women in particular locales. Mandatory or routine screening in conjunction with prenatal care puts women in the position of making a crisis decision about that pregnancy, which requires especially sensitive counseling beyond merely accepting the knowledge of serostatus. Some have argued that contact tracing is beneficial to women, since male partners are unlikely to inform women about their serostatus. But using contact tracing to offset women's existing problems with their male partners may render women more vulnerable to discrimination, especially if they cannot be integrated into a sensitive support network.

Contact tracing laws and programs must take into account the effects on women and couples when women learn about their male partners' risk behavior at the same time as discovering their diagnosis and the women's own serostatus. Because the impact of this series of discoveries may come with little preparation, the couple are likely to enter a crisis, which could result in domestic violence or dissolution of the relationship.

Programs might be better advised to put efforts into primary prevention rather than continuing to cope after the fact with infections that might have been averted through more aggressive risk-reduction campaigns. When contact tracing is used, counseling and support for seropositive women identified in this way must take into account the reality that women may have had little recognition of their partners' potential for being infected. Unlike individuals who go through some process to decide to be tested for HIV antibodies, those who are reached through contact tracing may be completely unprepared to make a knowledgeable decision about their readiness for testing and for coping with the results.

Overall, international and governmental attention to women's needs in the HIV epidemic have focused on macro-patterns rather than local variations. The general exclusion of women from political and planning processes has obscured the important local needs of women. To the extent that general, universally applicable programs have been developed (for example, the 'home party' model developed in the US and now used in many developing countries), there are rarely advocates for women in a position to modify policy and programs to accommodate local needs. Thus, women's issues have been simultaneously invisible and overgeneralized.

Projects for Women[1]

The issues faced by women with or at risk for HIV are multiple and locally specific. However, there are patterns in types of programs, with variations by region, culture, and women's socioeconomic status. Current programs generally fall into three broad categories — women's-group-based, family-based, and clinic-based — each with a somewhat different perception of and approach to the needs of seropositive women versus women perceived to be at risk but uninfected. The majority of current programs directed toward women are clinic-based, in part because the bulk of funding for women has gone to research programs in clinics or hospitals and in part because women primarily discover their HIV status in conjunction with undergoing some other form of health care, in relation to a pregnancy, STD care, or drug treatment.

Women's-Group-Based Projects

Women's-group-based programs generally do not make sharp distinctions between seropositive and seronegative women, and work equally with both groups. Women's-group-based programming is most concerned to prevent HIV infection among women, and to increase access to treatment and support services for already infected women. In addition, a small but vital network of groups by and for HIV seropositive women has emerged with a decided orientation toward women's groups.

Empower, in Bangkok, organizes a wide range of educational activities among sex workers. Recognizing that the major impediments to risk reduction among women are lack of information and inability to gain compliance on the part of male partners, Empower teaches literacy, 'life skills' (such as sewing, bookkeeping, finding and using social services), and self-esteem for women. By giving women concrete economic survival skills as well as confidence in their ability to make a living, Empower hopes to help women ensure safe sex compliance with clients and boyfriends or husbands. In addition, women teach each other about AIDS and HIV prevention, enhancing their communication skills and promoting the idea that women can be in control of information about self-protection.

South Carolina AIDS Education Network, in the US, operates from a beauty shop (Hair Ego) owned by SCAEN executive director DiAna DiAna. A member of the local black community, DiAna DiAna had become concerned about the lack of HIV prevention knowledge among her women clients. She began selling condoms from her shop, and quickly started informal safe sex education. As a volunteer support 'buddy' in the local people with AIDS project, DiAna DiAna was also aware of the gaps in support services available to women with AIDS and HIV. Hair Ego became the community's focal point for education and a center of support for already infected women. As enthusiasm for the project grew, clients of Hair Ego became involved in a wide range of AIDS support and education activities among themselves and with other members of their community.

Cefemina, a women's center in Costa Rica, began support and outreach activities for women involved in the national women's movement who were not being reached through government programs. Utilizing women volunteers supporting other infected or 'at risk' women, Cefemina organized a country-wide conference to discuss the needs of women with HIV and those who lacked risk-reduction education and support. The group uses an empowerment model that seeks to build women's skills and increase their participation in local decisionmaking and support activities in relation to HIV.

A wide range of locales, from inner-city minority communities in the US to linguistically diverse sections of Cape Verde and among drug injectors in Europe, use a 'home party' model to educate and support women at risk, and to inform those who may already be infected about their social service and medical options. In this model, a peer educator convenes already-existing informal groups of women (in neighborhoods or through churches or other community centers) who discuss their concerns about HIV infection and illness. These groups help women to collectively discover their needs, begin developing strategies to obtain care and achieve compliance with safe sex.

Women's-group-based projects tap existing support and information networks among women and help participants to identify existing or potential HIV-related concerns and develop realistic coping and risk-reduction strategies. Women-centered projects view women's subordinate social condition to be the root cause of women's HIV-related problems, and attempt to help women find self-empowering options for coping with problems.

Family-Centered Projects

Although focused on the individual person with AIDS, The AIDS Support Organization (TASO) in Uganda approaches women's HIV-related needs through their families. Because identified AIDS cases in urban Uganda typically include a man and one or more female partners and their children, TASO is able to effectively address many of women's needs for HIV-related counseling through supporting the women's families. TASO peer counselors, who are usually themselves persons with HIV/AIDS, replace or augment the roles in the family which have been disrupted by AIDS. Thus, TASO brings together a community of formerly unrelated family units for mutual support.

A similar program was developed from an evaluation of differences, by gender and ethnicity of expressed needs and use of services by clients of the AIDS Action Committee of Massachusetts, in the US. Women expressed greatest need for concrete financial, childcare, and housing support, while men expressed needs for money generally and for help coping with emotional problems. Men who did not have family members, especially women, needed more emotional and domestic assistance. Women needed less support for themselves, but greater support providing their traditional domestic and maternal services. The

AAC designed a project for 'lay caregivers' to help the people who were 'burning out' as a result of the burdens shifted onto them by the person with AIDS. Unlike most programs that offer support to the diagnosed person, this project was designed to support the other family members who had been taking care of the person with AIDS. The goal was to get help to family systems before the systems break down and reject the person with AIDS.

AIDS Prevention and Awareness in Native American Communities, a project of the Native American Women's Health Resource Center in South Dakota, US, also addresses women's needs through family and community. Here the woman is perceived to be an integral part of her community, and her needs for safe sex and for material and emotional support if infected are viewed as a community responsibility. Like projects in post-colonial countries, APANAC viewed the social causes of AIDS-related problems as stemming from the conflict between Western and non-Western attitudes. The project celebrates the traditional role played by homosexuals within the culture, thereby reducing the stigma attached to AIDS generally. The project works toward empowering women in their traditional roles as teachers and confidants by providing AIDS training and encouraging community conversation about the effects of AIDS and possibilities for re-uniting and strengthening local communities through their coping systems.

Family-based programs help women get needed resources and shift the burden of their illness and incapacity to perform their usual domestic tasks onto others. In some cases, volunteers step in to help; in other cases, traditional family and community coping strategies are strengthened and directed toward helping the woman with AIDS and her family.

Clinic-Based Programs

The bulk of existing programs for women are clinic-based. They range from informal 'drop-in' support groups with childcare that enable women to come and talk to formal and evaluated educational sessions designed to increase women's knowledge about AIDS and provide them with the basis for making future childbearing and treatment decisions. Many of these programs have grown out of maternal care units or women's health units of clinics and hospitals, and thus have some of the characteristics of women's-group-based programs.

Where women who join other projects are likely to have thought through their decision to become involved, women in clinic-based programs had been recruited through their medical providers, perhaps at the same time as or just after first learning of their serostatus. Thus, how women discover their serostatus is critical in designing counseling programs. In general, women discover their serostatus passively in one of three ways: after discovering that a male partner is infected, during their prenatal care process (Taylor, 1990), or through enrolment in a formal HIV-related study.

Women who had not previously identified themselves as 'at risk' will have considerably different needs than those who, for whatever reasons, have (correctly or not) identified risk and voluntarily sought testing or counseling. It is important to recognize that perception of risk may not correlate with objective risk or with serostatus. Perception of women's risk should not be tied to social roles such as 'sex worker' or 'sexually active', especially given that few women recognize the risk factors of their male partners. Educational programs which encourage testing, and therefore serve as a point of entry into test-based counseling systems, should avoid reinforcing social biases about 'who is at risk'.

The second route to knowledge of serostatus is through prenatal care programs which encourage testing. In this case, counseling protocols must recognize that the woman is faced with making crisis-oriented decisions about her current pregnancy. As discussed in earlier chapters, data from the US suggests a higher tendency to abort among women discovering their serostatus after becoming pregnant, but many of these same women carry a subsequent pregnancy to term. The reasons behind this series of decisions are complex: however, it is important for counselors to recognize that the immediate decision to avoid the possibilities of perinatal transmission may be re-evaluated by the woman later, when she has an opportunity to assess the decision in relation to cultural norms. The nuances involved in assessing the relative risk of such pregnancies, what will be valued as the morally 'right' choice, and whether women's self-esteem will be achieved by continuing (childrearing) or terminating (avoiding transmission) will depend on the evolving norms of the woman's family and community.

The third route to knowledge of serostatus is enrolment in targeted epidemiological studies, usually ones initiated through drug treatment centers or among relatively organized groups of prostitutes contacted through STD clinics. While certain groups of people undergoing testing — middle-class attenders at anonymous testing sites and members of organized gay communities — may have considerable knowledge about HIV and access to community-wide debates about testing and its relevance, the vast majority of high risk-women are tested and receive results with little understanding of the ramifications of testing and virtually no one to talk to. Some programs, especially those among sex workers, have consciously developed intra-group interaction and support processes which can be ongoing, tapping gossip networks and informal leaders to introduce and circulate knowledge and challenge evolving norms.

It is important to recognize that women who discover their serostatus through involvement in research studies will have different needs than women learning through prenatal care or through diagnosis of their partner. Study participants always have mixed motives for involvement — desire for self-knowledge, benefits of adjunct health care, altruism. Especially in settings where research protocols are a major method for discovering one's serostatus or for easily obtaining coordinated care, the desire to undergo testing may overshadow acquisition of knowledge about AIDS or development of risk-reduction plans. While the technical information needed by women in research protocols may be the same, their reasons for involvement suggest the need for more tailored counseling or support programs.

Institutional Changes in International Projects

Coordination of HIV Projects for Women

Currently, international organizations and the World Health Organization contain many departments and programs which are directly or tangentially dealing with issues affecting women, resulting in both duplication of efforts and gaps in planning. International AIDS-related organizations and organizations which serve women generally should establish specific posts designed to coordinate women's health, educational, and social support needs in relationship to HIV. Efforts to 'fold in' AIDS programming with existing, related projects may sometimes be the most efficient mechanism for dealing with service delivery; however, the substantial gender-related differences in HIV issues suggest that we have not yet developed adequately conceived and designed programs for women to integrate into other forms of health and education delivery. In addition, while much has been accomplished in the past few years in terms of program modification, addressing women's ongoing needs and coordinating future programs and research require the continuity and visibility of designated posts.

Unfortunately, the Global Programme on AIDS has moved toward decentralization in the last three years, a move which may be premature, especially in regard to the needs of developing countries. Many national programs in developing countries, especially in the African Region, have worked closely with GPA to develop programs for women, and these regional and national offices can continue to play a crucial role in coordinating and gathering information about activities for women at the local level. Projects involving cooperation between developed and developing countries have produced viable projects for women, a decentralization solution which promises to distribute the financial burden and technical support for AIDS-related projects across wealthier countries. However, this complex of national, non-governmental, and World Health Organization programming brings mixed political agendas, making it difficult in many cases to actually respond to local needs, which are often quite straightforward. At least in relation to gender-specific programming, there continues to be a need for some form of international coordination and for interconnection of national AIDS programs in order to disseminate existing findings and information about women's needs and to suggest program modifications which will address women's needs.

The current activities to link NGOs and create closer ties with national organizations must address women's issues more intensively and proactively. At this time, services for and programs by gay men, sex workers, and male persons with HIV/ AIDS far outnumber those for and by women. This is in part due to the long time it has taken to help women and service providers recognize the existence and needs of women with HIV. Equally significant, however, are the greater structural power and access of men; as detailed above, women have great difficulty organizing themselves and articulating their needs because of cultural and structural impediments. NGO efforts must become proactive in relation to women's needs, recognizing that women have different kinds of organizational and technical skills which may make it difficult for small, local groups to fit into existing funding models. There is a tendency to view the ability to apply for small grants as a benchmark in the growth and stabilization of volunteer/NGO groups. However, local women's projects may be so organically developed and so accustomed to operating without hope of external support that they do not recognize themselves as an 'NGO'. Programs which offer small grants to NGOs must actively solicit and support small, community-based women's programs.

Program Development and Research

Despite the dramatic increase in papers on women's issues presented at recent international conferences on AIDS, there continues to be a lack of systematic and comparable information on HIV and women. There are exciting and promising projects underway in many locales that have yet to be documented in a way that makes even cursory evaluation possible. KABPs on attitudes toward sexuality and condom use are not sufficient for program development as they neither take into account the cultural rationales for patterns of behavior nor the existing social mechanisms for coping, which may help or impede risk reduction programs. Research needs must not overshadow innovations on the local level, which tend to occur organically, but prospective, qualitative analysis of existing and new programs is essential.

Multidisciplinary, innovative research on community- and gender-specific modes of coping and effects of crisis must be undertaken to inform planners about the possibilities for long-term adaptation to the needs of risk reduction and care. Such research must identify existing traditional practices that could be readily adapted to incorporate HIV education, counseling, and care components. In addition, HIV is significantly affecting and affected by traditional gender and social roles; as suggested above — especially in relation to migration — breakdown in traditional gender roles improves the status of some women, but increases the poverty and vulnerability of other women. More egalitarian family structures may enhance the ability of women to ensure safe sexual practices and more evenly allocate provision of primary care, but it also lessens the advantages of marriage for men, which may result in increasing poverty for women. While these topics have been researched in some contexts, there should be some research that at least schematizes the dynamic social processes accompanying the reality of coping with HIV and the side-effects of risk-reduction campaigns.

In addition, research on the economic status and production role of women in developing countries should assess the effects of potential increases in morbidity and mortality of women due to HIV. Likewise, the role of community-controlled HIV programs which also help women gain new skills should be analyzed for economic feasibility.

Evaluation of current HIV counseling and education programs for women should not only include data on behavior change and knowledge acquisition, but should also be evaluated for their capacity to enhance women's self-esteem, skills, and participation in family and community decisionmaking. While attitude, knowledge, and behavior change are important, they only address the short-term problems of prevention. Only larger changes in women's social status will finally enable a change in transmission patterns.

As I have suggested throughout, women's needs are on one level universal, and on another highly locally specific. To date, women involved in research, planning, program design, and local organizing, and especially women living with HIV, have had relatively few opportunities to meet, pool their knowledge, and evaluate the similarities and differences in their local experiences. Conferences specifically on women's HIV-related issues globally, including researchers, policymakers, and women living with HIV from countries with high, medium, and low prevalence could help consolidate information and experience and could also help develop the core components of a forward-looking plan to meet the multiple needs of women during the HIV pandemic.

Education and Training

Women lack structural power on all levels of health research, policy, and program implementation. While grass-roots projects may be successful, there is an overall, structural incapacity to pursue extension and development of those programs to other cities or countries. Because local women's empowerment may seem threatening to municipal or local officials, organizations like the Global Programme on AIDS and the Red Cross, which have been effective in persuading countries to initiate programs in the areas of sex work, street children, and community-based care, should use their influence to stimulate interest in women's projects. Programs for women are often difficult to start and maintain: existing AIDS-related international organizations are in an ideal situation to identify existing programs and potential sites for implementing pilot projects that develop existing programs and traditional women's networks to provide HIV counseling and support. While maternal and child health and family planning projects have moved toward incorporating HIV education and counseling into existing programs, these efforts address women's needs largely from the standpoint of institutions. Efficient use of community resources and the crucial long-term empowerment of women locally require initiation of HIV projects developed and managed by women. But these programs must also be sensitively designed: 'empowerment' may have different meanings in different settings, requiring close attention to the social and power structures in local communities.

Planners should assume that indigenous systems for information and support provision exist. Counseling should be construed in the broadest possible context, including formal, clinically-based models, traditional modes of emotional and social support, and emerging self-help forms (such as TASO in Uganda) which weave together local, traditional support systems with the principles and concerns developing within the international PLWA movements.

Improved Understanding of Lesbian Sexuality

Many of the studies on self-identified lesbians are crude, but several elements recur. First, many lesbians acknowledge a theoretical risk for the behaviors in which they engage and yet do not elect to use practices to reduce risk. This may mean that lesbians perceive a technical risk, but do not believe anyone they have sex with will be seropositive. There is also apparently little concern for eliminating other possible STDs which would be a secondary benefit of adopting barrier methods.

Second, large-sample quantitative studies suggest that drug-injecting lesbians and bisexual women are exposed and subsequently infected at much higher rates than their heterosexual peers. This is another area urgently in need of qualitative research to discover the relationship between conducting an alternative sexual lifestyle and increased exposure to HIV. Although all of these studies suggest that more education needs to be targeted to women who have sex with women, it is still unclear what to say: apparently, self-identified and study-identified lesbians and bisexual women have the same general information as everyone else; simply routing more information is likely to be ineffective. Given that it is unlikely that female-to-female practices are a major source of their infection, 'lesbian' pamphlets may once again backfire. On the other hand, there is a growing body of knowledge about female-to-female transmission, which should be included in any materials directed to women.

There is an urgent need for intervention/research projects which undertake to describe the real lives of the women who appear as statistics in the drug-related studies. Qualitative studies have incidental reports on lesbian participants and quantitative studies may have unreported data on female-to-female sexual practices. An immediate first step would be to assemble and reanalyze all direct and incidental existing data and then pursue more detailed investigation. In addition, both programs directed at drug injectors and programs that interface with the more visible core of the lesbian community must initiate more active cross-education about the life contexts which seem to put more disenfranchised women in a situation of increased risk.

The schizophrenic approach which pits a class-distinct group of lesbians who proclaim their distance from any HIV risk against the increasing number of lesbians and bisexual women who are seropositive due to drug injection, sex with men, or possibly sex with women only defeats efforts to get a sensitive response from researchers, clinics and AIDS service organizations. Continuing the divisive split between women who fear major female to female transmission and those who are unconvinced of any risk ignores the life experience of lesbians who have not been incorporated into the economic, social, and political community; the latter could be emotionally sustaining and even life-saving. There is currently enough information to be realistic about the low feasibility of woman-to-woman trans-mission without turning activist attention away from providing advice on degrees of risk and risk reduction or from the needs of lesbian and bisexual women who have contracted HIV through 'non-lesbian' activities.

There have been numerous studies of why gay and heter-osexual men, heterosexual women, and gay and straight couples do not practice safe sex in the face of their own perception of risk. Information from these has proved crucial in the design of second-phase education material which helps well-informed individuals develop strategies for pursuing safer sex and can help whole communities move toward safe sex and safe drug use norms. This kind of study is essential now for determining what to do next to help self-identified lesbians and bisexual women. The apparently significant and intransigent lesbian dislike of dental dams (Hunter *et al.*, 1992) seems to have stopped the process in its tracks. The dislike of technique may mask a variety of other issues, such as a history of sexual abuse or having felt that a lesbian lifestyle meant an end to worry about birth control and sexual health. The apparent reason for not moving past dislike of technique is a perception that lesbians' likelihood of contracting STDs and HIV through sexual activity is low. While this may remain true for HIV (hepatitis and herpes are much more easily transmitted), this is not a sufficient reason to avoid developing better technologies for improving the general sexual health of lesbians and bisexual women.

Counseling

In addition to assessing how and why women seek testing, counseling programs should have a good understanding of local norms of who is expected to speak to whom about sexuality. There is a common and erroneous assumption about many cultures that 'sex is not discussed'. However, it is actually rare to find cultures or groups where there is no discussion of sexuality — if only under the guise of advice about marriage and childbearing. Counseling should use people and settings similar to those women are used to for discussing sexuality.

Counselors should help women identify their existing support systems. Many women do not believe they can get support from their families or their spouses' families. Counselors should work with clients to determine how extended family members can be mobilized to help them. Educating families and communities is an effective way of aiding individual clients.

Counselors may also find that self-help projects are the most beneficial form of longer-term support for women living with HIV. With minimal additional training (most clients are already 'experts' on HIV), women living with HIV can be extremely effective educators for everyone and sensitive counselors to other seropositive women. Empowerment of women living with HIV can help offset the tendency to overmedicalize their situation and decrease the stigma surrounding AIDS by enhancing their status as a source of information and support within their communities.

Counselors seem to believe that the most controversial issue facing the seropositive woman is whether to have children. While it is true that in almost every culture, women's worth is equated with their childbearing capacity, the problem of the ethics of childbearing seems sometimes to overwhelm counselors' ability to discern the complexity of issues concerning the status, care, and self-perceptions of seropositive women. Many cultures place tremendous pressure on women and couples to have children. This is viewed as the couple's contribution to the community, proof of the man's masculinity, the sole opportunity for the woman to be involved in the social world. Choosing *not* to have children eliminates a major route to self-esteem, social connectedness, and power for women and their male partners.

While the tragedy of a child born with HIV is compelling, women's childbearing decisions must be placed in the larger context. Women worldwide are choosing to take the risk of bearing an HIV-seropositive child for a variety of personal and socially influenced reasons. While it is extremely important for counselors to help women and their male partners assess the risks of bearing an infected child, it is equally important to help the women determine other means of achieving self-esteem and social connectedness if they choose not to have children.

Counselors should recognize that women living with HIV are extremely concerned about the welfare of their children, even to the point of avoiding clinics for fear that the children will be taken away. Counselors should help women develop plans for how they will care for their children, how they will cope with the possible illness affecting their children, how their families and communities will help them, and how they will support and care for their children if they themselves become sick.

In some cultures, bearing an infected child may seem cruel, and a woman who takes this risk might be considered irrational simply because she desires a child in these circumstances. Counselors must back away from their own assumptions and try to understand the specific reasons a woman has for pursuing a pregnancy. Male partners and other family members may be important influences on women's decisions. Women may fear direct reprisals, or they may simply expect to take directions from family or husband. In cases where a woman does not want a pregnancy but is under pressure from other family members, it may be necessary to incorporate those people into the counseling process. Overemphasis on the event of childbearing, and exclusive focus on the woman may obscure other significant issues and interrelationships within families and communities.

Clearly, feminist activists the world over have challenged the cultural norms which accord women status based on their children. While it may be impossible to overcome broad sexism of this kind in an individual case, it is critical for counselors to recognize that the participants in a childbearing decision may be acting from such beliefs even when they do not intend to. If seropositive women choose not to have children (which seems to be the barely unstated wish of most counseling programs), they must not only be supported for avoiding 'vertical transmission' but their potential real loss of status and loss of self-esteem must be addressed. Similarly, if women choose to have children, the issues that arise from caring for potentially infected children and from watching their own health decline must be addressed in the context of women's place in families and communities that pressure women to have children.

There is a good chance that safe sex or birth control have already been a problem, and in the case of any woman infected through unprotected intercourse, she has clearly not been able to effect her wishes to practice safe sex. People who know they are infected may decide not to practice safe sex with partners who are also infected, believing that it is 'already too late'. It is important to emphasize that subsequent reinfection, or infection with other STDs, can worsen the progression of HIV illnesses. Although both partners are under the stress of coping with being seropositive, condom use should be promoted as a means of staying asymptomatic or slowing progression by avoiding additional infections.

Counselors should help women strategize for discussing changes in sexual behavior with their partners. Sex can become the focus for other frustrations or struggles, further disempowering women from maintaining their health. Work with couples and self-help groups can provide excellent long-term support for women attempting to change their own and their partners' sexual practices.

Women living with HIV feel isolated and unworthy of concern, and find it difficult to discuss their concerns even with their friends and family. Especially in sexual encounters, women do not feel they have the right to ask for safe sex. One reason why women express such extreme concern for their children is because they do not believe they are themselves worthy of support or assistance.

A major role of the counselor is to help women improve their status, including their belief in their own worth. All the decisions and issues an HIV-seropositive woman will have to address, including those concerning childbearing, seeking medical treatment, and practicing safe sex, will be strongly influenced by her feeling of self-worth. Counselors can help women feel more positive, but longer-term changes in women's immediate environment and culture are necessary. Counselors should expand their concept of their role by encouraging women to start self-help projects or by referring women to already existing projects.

Self-help projects around HIV/AIDS education and support can be doubly helpful for women. Not only can women speak publicly about their illness and find direct avenues of support, they can also gain skills and confidence that come from being a recognized teacher and helper. Involvement in education and support projects will also provide a new sense of belonging. It is important for people living with HIV *and* their community to see that they are positive and contributing members.

Counseling can play an important role in supporting seropositive women both through the crisis of diagnosis and in their ongoing decisionmaking processes. While the medical and crisis-related needs of men and women may be similar, women's lower social status makes it difficult for them to gain support for crucial decisions. Counseling can help women both immediately and in the longer-term by taking their special concerns seriously and from the women's own perspective, and by advocating for women with other family or community members.

But while much attention internationally has been focused on counseling, planners should recognize that counseling is fundamentally an Anglo/American concept. Most other cultures lack the social role and the concept of designated individuals who confidentially provide advice, information, and support. Cultures with strong extended family or tight community infrastructures generally have a 'counseling' system which designates particular classes of people (for example, grand-mothers, or religious or political leaders) as those who serve as the repository for folk and technical wisdom. In other cultures, there are age-linked structures which determine who is allowed to speak about sensitive issues. Assessment of existing support and education structures should be sensitive to how gender and age structures affect transfer of information and mobilization of coping systems.

It is true that the concepts of community or grass-roots organizing are adaptable in most settings, including post-colonial societies where traditional infrastructures may have been diminished without a corollary increase in state-mediated services, self-help is also a culture-bound concept. The idea of 'self-help' only arises once substantial institution-mediated services ('other-help') exist. For example, the PLWA movement model with its ideas of living with dignity and hope have been successfully adapted in the TASO project in Uganda. However, it should be noted that the PLWA movement has thus far centered chiefly on the issues and needs faced by men, or by families contacted through an infected male member. This model may not be applicable to systems in which women are the identified clients, or which are attempting to reach out to women not previously served by health-related services used to cope with HIV.

Institutionally-based counseling programs (including those using out-clinics or visiting teams) should be designed to provide the full range of information and service referral for women, consistent with regional, cultural, economic, religious, linguistic, or other differences. In many cases, institutional programs will continue to serve as a central point for information and referral. While community members may become involved, such projects are not truly 'grass-roots' since community members must evolve their ideas within institutional constraints.

It is crucial to understand the difference between institution-mediated services and those evolving from existing social structures, even though in many cases the two forms of programming will converge at some point. Since women have traditionally provided the bulk of both primary care and emotional support, priority should be given to developing existing resources among women or initiating programs which enable such networks to remain intact. While it may be necessary to provide institutionally-mediated services, or technical assistance in supporting traditional structures, creating dependence on institutions can cause traditional systems to atrophy, resulting in dramatic, potentially irreversible damage to social structures.

Finally, the complexity of gender and social roles, and their determinative effects on risk reduction, care, and decision-making may make it impossible to develop a single prototype for women's counseling, especially in relation to childbearing. A considerable amount of technically correct material exists, but the process through which such material and information is introduced and used will be highly variable. However, it is possible to develop a series of questions and issues to aid in local and possibly regional programs.

Looking Ahead

Women's health needs have been identified as an overlooked aspect of national health plans. Despite the efforts of the Decade for Women, the crisis in women's health has actually increased in the past two decades due to worldwide recession which has left women among the poorest of the poor. Now, the HIV epidemic threatens to throw poor women and women in developing nations even deeper into poverty. Women's lives are at stake; the lives of children, families, and even entire countries — in places where women are a major part of agricultural production — are in jeopardy. Massive changes in conceptualization and planning for women must occur; short-term crisis plans must take into account the long-term need to lift women out of the conditions which create their poverty and the great morbidity and mortality resulting from AIDS. Although this is a big order for countries with already strained budgets, there are important existing projects which are low cost and involve women in their own and their children's health, education and care. These programs should be formally evaluated and implemented in other locales with similar needs and informal resources.

Projects start from a variety of places — hospitals, clinics, women's groups, churches — for historically specific reasons (usually a particular death or community experience). The autonomy and special reasons for the origin of each program should be respected, because it is the personal investments in such projects which create the energy and desire to pursue them. However, when possible, programs should be linked in order to avoid duplication of energy or lack of attention to other people's needs. Collaboration between diverse projects creates better mutual understanding of the diverse needs of people affected by HIV, and may help local groups present a more coherent face and long-range plans to funding or government agencies. Empowering those most directly affected by HIV, but especially those who have experienced historic patterns of discrimination and who live in economic, social, and political systems which devalue their contributions is an essential component of all HIV-related programs and plans. While groups have differing interests and perspectives on the causes and solutions to the epidemic, these differences need not conflict if the common, systemic impediments to services and humane treatment are identified.

Developing locally successful prevention and care projects will almost inevitably become political: the crucial battle is to acknowledge the dimensions of varying political agendas and form solid and meaningful alliances among those suffering from social discrimination and the resultant poor management of health promotion systems.

Notes

1   The information on specific projects comes primarily from conversations I had with the organizers at conferences and at meetings attempting to coordinate programming concerning women. For further information, see Center for Women Policy Studies (1990) and The ACT UP/New York Women and AIDS Book Group (1990).

Chapter 7

Epilogue

As promised, this book complicates the idea of 'woman' and her needs in the context of the HIV pandemic. Based in US epidemiology and its social and cultural concepts of gender and sexuality, the categories for counting those affected in the epidemic are deeply culture-bound. Policy and research, too, have not stretched very far from their original, disciplinary conceptions of 'women', if women indeed figured in their work at all. The US media recycled their own constructions of women, altering and complementing those already instrinsic to the science they reported and those already present in the minds of the public they addressed.

It is the logic of various definitions of 'woman', and the ways they are used in HIV media coverage, policy, education, and activism, that organizes this volume. This is not an intellectual exercise in category dissection, but an attempt to suggest where and how more successful coalitions can be formed, and an attempt to offer some framework for acknowledging the differences in strategy which do and will continue to occur among those of us committed to improving women's lives, especially in the urgent context of the HIV epidemic. With better ways to proceed, we might be more cognizant of the power of the categories we inherit and perhaps a little more sanguine about whether and how we can intervene in them. We may be better able to treat women's needs in the cultural contexts in which they arise, understanding, challenging, and reforming the working hypotheses about women in particular locales.

The interrelationship between women's health and women's status is complex and paradoxical. On one hand, there is a need to remove institutional, cultural, social, and economic barriers to women's participation in the family and society and access to resources. This requires gender-blind programming. On the other hand, women lag behind in important skills and in their sense of social worth, so that special programs must be instituted, perhaps for some time, in order to help women acquire the skills and self-confidence to participate in their world more actively. Finally, women have been the chief providers of critical primary health and mental health care, and should be recognized for their crucial role, again requiring information and consciousness-raising campaigns which highlight women as special contributors. Because of these paradoxical needs, two strategies for HIV counseling and prevention with HIV seropositive and other women must be pursued. One strategy, generally, will seek to eliminate discrimination against women in social, economic, and political structures and attitudes in order to enable women to pursue risk-reduction and coping strategies. The second will seek to empower women on the local and family level in order to help them gain skills, confidence, and support in effecting risk reduction and making wise choices about their HIV-related care.

Most importantly, however, activists and planners must understand the interrelationship betweeen women's special issues and the special issues faced by other groups, especially gay men. Unfortunately, the increase in attention to women's concerns has sometimes come at the cost of pushing the issues of gay men aside, resulting in both 'de-gaying' and de-funding crucial existing projects. As I have suggested throughout, the linkage between AIDS and the gay community created a broad perception that HIV was related to deviance, and much of the conceptualization and policy surrounding AIDS has been highly stigmatizing. Though correct in technical terms, the effort to pursuade people that 'AIDS does not discriminate' and that 'anyone can get AIDS' mainstreamed the epidemic in complicated ways: the attempt to hail members of the 'general population' — especially women — came at the cost of discontinued education of gay men. The split between the mainstream and the supposedly deviant communities which underwrote AIDS education and information from early in the epidemic continues to make it difficult to design campaigns and programs that address both gay men and women. In the past few years, longstanding activists in gay communities have expressed anger over the new emphasis on women's concerns, especially given that, at least in developed countries, gay men continue to be a major affected group. However frustrating, the shift in funding and ideological priorities is not merely an effect of homophobia nor a testament to the success of women's rights, but a result of the original misconception of the epidemic as primarily affecting members of a deviant subgroup. Having constituted the epidemiological landscape through this split, education overemphasized self-identification with socially stigmatized behavior. The media have attempted to retreat from their original misrepresentation of the epidemic by 'de-gaying' AIDS, and shifting their focus to the need to 'protect women'. But protecting 'women' is another subtle ruse, because AIDS discourse does not, finally, allow anyone to be 'innocent'.

The category 'innocence' is largely a place holder, a way of imagining someone else who would be less responsible than the group or individual actually under discussion. Media accounts may use women to fill this role in juxtaposition to bisexual men. But as suggested in Chapter Five, the same media portray the individual woman who actually contracts HIV from such a man as 'loose' or as a dupe who is unable to distinguish 'real' men from those who may have contracted HIV from another man. Innocence only exists in the abstract: the huge stigma of contracting HIV continues to make every individual person living with the virus suspected of having 'done something wrong'.

This insistent blaming of the person who has contracted HIV continues in large part because the range and complex social meanings of human sexual behavior are poorly documented and even less well understood. Homosexuality is widely marginalized and even criminalized, seriously hampering AIDS education and safer sex campaigns. But *heterosexuality* has not been taken seriously in the AIDS epidemic either: sex is supposed to be practiced in the confines of a monogamous relationship, legitimated by the state and/or religion. Sexualities and sexual health needs that fall outside the married couple have been ignored at best. The failure to take heterosexual patterns and heterosexual safer sex seriously has weighed most heavily on women, who are already socially, culturally, politically, and economically disadvantaged by the institutions designed to support and enforce heterosexuality. Women have long been disenfranchised by social and medical systems; because AIDS is still understood through the lens of deviance, women living with HIV will continue to be the last served.

Bibliography

ABRAHAMSON, PAUL R. and HERDT, GILBERT (1990) 'The Assessment of Sexual Practices Relevant to the Transmission of AIDS: A Global Perspective', *Journal of Sex Research*, 27/2, May.

THE ACT UP/NEW YORK WOMEN AND AIDS BOOK GROUP (1990) *Women, AIDS and Activism*, Boston, South End Press.

AFRICA RIGHTS MONITOR (1990) No. 16, *Africa Today*, 37/1.

ALEXANDER, NANCY J. *et al.* (1990) *Heterosexual Transmission of AIDS*, New York, Wiley-Liss.

ALMA, W. (1986) 'Psycho-Social Problems of Migrants', in *Migration and Health*, Geneva, WHO.

ANDERSON, J. *et al.* (1989) 'Knowledge of HIV Serostatus and Pregnancy Decisions', paper presented at Fifth International Conference on AIDS, Montreal.

ANKRAH, E. M. *et al.* (1992) 'Rural and Urban Mobility and Attendant Sexual Behavior', paper presented at Eighth International Conference on AIDS, Amsterdam.

ANTONIO, GENE (1986) *The AIDS Cover-Up? The Real and Alarming Facts about AIDS*, San Francisco, Ignatius Press.

BAILEY, PATRICIA *et al.* (1992) 'Heterogeneity Among Commercial Sex Workers and Commonalities of Condom Use', paper presented at Eighth International Conference on AIDS, Amsterdam.

BELLIS, DAVID J. (1990) 'Fear of AIDS and Risk Reduction Among Heroin-Addicted Female Street Prostitutes: Personal Interviews with 72 Southern California Subjects', *Journal of Alcohol and Drug Education*, 35/3, Spring.

BEOKU-BETTS, JOSEPHINE (1990) 'Agricultural Development in Sierra Leone: Implications for Rural Women in the Aftermath of the Women's Decade', *Africa Today*, 37/1.

BERNARD, MARINA and MCKEGANEY, NEIL (1992) 'Risk Behaviors Among a Sample of Male Clients of Female Prostitutes', paper presented at Eighth International Conference on AIDS, Amsterdam.

BEVIER, PAMELA *et al.* (1992) 'Women Who Have Sex with Women and Multiple Risks for HIV at a New York City STD Clinic', paper presented at Eighth International AIDS Conference, Amsterdam.

BOUE, F. *et al.* (1990) 'Risks for HIV 1 Perinatal Transmission Vary with the Mother's Stage of Infection', paper presented at International AIDS Conference, San Francisco.

Bibliography

BRANCH FOR THE ADVANCEMENT OF WOMEN (1989) 'AIDS and Its Effects on the Advancement of Women', Women 2000, Vienna, Centre for Social Development and Humanitarian Concerns.

BRANDT, ALLAN (1985) *No Magic Bullet*, London, Oxford University Press.

BROCKETT, LINDA *et al.* (1992) 'HIV/AIDS Prevention Targeting Asian Prostitution in Sydney — A Cultural Perspective', paper presented at Eighth International Conference on AIDS, Amsterdam.

BRONFMAN, MARIO *et al.* (1992) 'Sexual Habits of Temporary Mexican-Migrants to the United States of America: Risk Practices for HIV Infection', paper presented at Eighth International Conference on AIDS, Amsterdam.

CAMPBELL, CAROLE E. (1991) 'Prostitution, AIDS, and Preventive Health Behavior', *Social Science and Medicine*, 32/12.

CAMPBELL, IAN D. and WILLIAMS, GLEN (1990) *AIDS Management: An Integrated Approach*, Strategies for Hope Series, No. 3, London, ActionAid.

CENTER FOR WOMEN POLICY STUDIES (1990) *The Guide to Resources on Women and AIDS*, Washington, DC.

CHU, SUSAN *et al.* (1990) 'Epidemiology of Reported Cases of AIDS in Lesbians, United States 1980–89', *American Journal of Public Health*.

COHEN, JUDITH *et al.* (1992) 'Different Types of Prostitution Show Wide Variation in HIV and Other Sexually-Transmitted Disease Risk', paper presented at Eighth International Conference on AIDS, Amsterdam.

COHEN, ROBERTA and WISEBERG, LAURIE S. (1990) *Double Jeopardy — Threat to Life and Human Rights: Discrimination against Persons with AIDS*, Cambridge, MA, Human Rights Internet.

COLEMAN, SAMUEL (1981) 'The Cultural Context of Condom Use in Japan', *Studies in Family Planning 12/1*, January.

COWAN, JANE E. *et al.* (1990) 'Reproductive Choices of Women At Risk of HIV Infection', paper presented at Sixth International Conference on AIDS, San Francisco.

DAY, SOPHIE *et al.* (1992) 'Commercial Sex and HIV Risk: Male Parters of Female Sex Workers', paper presented at Eighth International Conference on AIDS, Amsterdam.

DE BRUYN, MARIA (1992) 'Women and AIDS in Developing Countries', *Social Science and Medicine*, 32/3.

DE CASO, L. E. *et al.* (1992) 'Qualitative Analysis and Linguistic Methodology for the Design of Education Material for AIDS Prevention Among Commercial Sex Workers', paper presented at Eighth International Conference on AIDS, Amsterdam.

DE GRAAF, RON *et al.* (1992) 'Heterosexual Prostitution Networks in the Netherlands and Britain', paper presented at Eighth International Conference on AIDS, Amsterdam.

DE ZALDUANDO, BARBARA O. (1991) 'Prostitution Viewed Cross-Culturally: Toward Recontextualizing Sex Work in AIDS Intervention Research', *Journal of Sex Research*, 28/2, May.

DORFMAN, LORI E., DERISH, PAMELA A. and COHEN, JUDITH B. (1992) 'Hey Girlfriend: An Evaluation of AIDS Prevention Among Women in the Sex Industry', *Health Education Quarterly*, 19/1. Spring.

EHRENREICH, BARBARA (1983) *The Hearts of Men*, Garden City, NY, Doubleday.

EHRENREICH, BARBARA and EHRENREICH, JOHN (1971) *The American Health Empire: Report of Health PAC*, New York, Vintage.

EHRENREICH, BARBARA and ENGLISH, DEIRDRE (1973) *Complaints and Disorders: The Sexual Politics of Sickness*, Westbury, NY, Feminist Press.

EHRENREICH, BARBARA, STOLLARD, KAREN and SKLAR, HOLLY (1983) *Poverty and the American Dream: Women and Children First*, Boston, South End Press.

ELIFSON, KIRK *et al.* (1992) 'HIV Seroprevalence and Risk Factors Among Clients of Male and Female Prostitutes', paper presented at Eighth International Conference on AIDS, Amsterdam.

ERICKSON, J. R. *et al.* (1992) 'Risk for HIV Among Homeless Male and Female Intravenous Drug Users (IDUs) in the United States', paper presented at Eighth International Conference on AIDS, Amsterdam.

ESTEBANEZ, PILAR *et al.* (1992) 'HIV Prevalence and Risk Factors in Spanish Prostitutes', paper presented at Eighth International Conference on AIDS, Amsterdam.

FERGUSON, JANE (1987) 'Reproductive Health of Adolescent Girls', *World Health Statistics Quarterly*, 40/3.

FLEMING, ALAN (1988) 'Prevention of Transmission of HIV by Blood Transfusion in Developing Countries', paper presented at Global Impact of AIDS Conference, London, 8–10 March.

FRIEDMAN, SAMUEL R. *et al.* (1992) 'HIV Seroconversion Among Street-Recruited Drug Injectors Who Have Sex with Women', paper presented at Eighth International Conference on AIDS, Amsterdam.

GALLOIS, CYNTHIA *et al.* (1990) 'Preferred Strategies for Safe Sex: Relation to Past and Actual Behavior Among Sexually Active Men and Women', paper presented at International AIDS Conference, San Francisco.

GASHAU, WADZANI *et al.* (1992) 'Awareness Regarding AIDS and HIV Seroprevalence in Nigerian Long Distance Truck Drivers', paper presented at Eighth International Conference on AIDS, Amsterdam.

GILMORE, NORBERT *et al.* (1992) 'A Worldwide Survey Of HIV/AIDS-Related Entry Restrictions', paper presented at Eighth International Conference on AIDS, Amsterdam.

HAOUR-KNIPE, MARY (1992) 'EC Concerted Action "Assessment of the AIDS/HIV Prevention Strategies": Migrants and Travellers', paper presented at Eighth International Conference on AIDS, Amsterdam.

HASSIG, SUSAN *et al.* (1989) 'Contraceptive Utilization and Reproductive Desires in a Group of HIV-Positive Women in Kinshasa', paper presented at Fifth International Conference on AIDS, Montreal.

HAWKES, S. J. *et al.* (1992) 'A Study of the Prevalence of HIV Infection and Associated Risk Factors in International Travellers', paper presented at Eighth International Conference on AIDS, Amsterdam.

HENDRICKS, AART (1990) *AIDS and Mobility*, Copenhagen, WHO Regional Office.

HEROLD, EDWARD *et al.* (1992) 'Canadian Tourists and Sexual Relationships', paper presented at Eighth International Conference on AIDS, Amsterdam.

HOLMAN, SUSAN *et al.* (1989) 'Women Infected with Human Immunodeficiency Virus: Counseling and Testing During Pregnancy', *Seminars in Perinatology*, 13/1, February.

HOUSE-MIDAMBA, BESSIE (1990) 'The United Nations Decade: Political Empowerment or Increased Marginalization for Kenyan Women?', *Africa Today*, 37/1.

HUGHES, VERONICA *et al.* (1992) 'Perceptions in the Use of Lubricants Among Prostitutes', paper presented at Eighth International Conference on AIDS, Amsterdam.

HUNTER, JOYCE *et al.* (1992) 'Sexual and Substance Abuse Acts that Place Lesbians at Risk for HIV', paper presented at Eighth International Conference on AIDS, Amsterdam.

HUTCHINSON, MARGARET and KURTH, ANN (1991) 'I Need to Know that I have a Choice: A Study of Women, HIV, and Reproductive Decision-Making', *AIDS Patient Care*, 5/1, February.

IARDINO, R. *et al.* (1992) 'Potential Routes of HIV Transmission Among Women', paper presented at the *Eighth International Conference on AIDS*, Amsterdam.

Bibliography

JUAREZ, I. *et al.* (1992) 'Prevalence and Determinants of HIV and Other STDs in a Population of Female Commercial Sex Workers in Mexico City', paper presented at Eighth International Conference on AIDS, Amsterdam.

KANE, STEPHANIE (1990) 'AIDS, Addiction and Condom Use: Sources of Sexual Risk for Heterosexual Women', *The Journal of Sex Research*, 27/3. August.

KANE, STEPHANIE (1989) 'HIV, Heroin and Heterosexual Relations', *Social Science and Medicine*, 32/9.

KAPLAN, MARK *et al.* (1989) 'Pregnancy Arising in HIV Infected Women While Being Repetitively Counseled About "Safe Sex"', paper presented at Fifth International Conference on AIDS, Montreal.

KIEREINI, EUNICE MURINGO (1990) 'Women and Children in Africa: AIDS Impact', Keynote Address at the Sixth International Conference on AIDS, San Francisco.

KUMARESAN, GANESAN *et al.* (1992) 'Safer Sex for Truckers: Puzhal Tamilnadu', paper presented at Eighth International Conference on AIDS, Amsterdam.

LEVINE, STEPHEN B. and AGLE, DAVID P. (1987) 'Intimacy, Sexuality and Hemophilia', New York, Hemophilia Foundation.

MAGANA, J. RAUL (1991) 'Sex, Drugs and HIV: An Ethnographic Approach', *Social Science and Medicine*, 33/1.

MASON, PATRICK, OLSON, ROBERTA and PARISH, KATHY (1988) 'AIDS, Hemophilia, and Prevention Efforts Within a Comprehensive Care Program', *American Psychologist*, 43/11.

MASTERS, WILLIAM H., JOHNSON, VIRGINIA E. and KOLODNY, ROBERT C. (1988) *Crisis: Heterosexual Behaviour in the Age of AIDS*, London, Weidenfeld and Nicolson.

MCKEGANEY, NEIL and BARNARD, MARINA (1992) 'Female Prostitution and HIV Infection in Glasgow', paper presented at Eighth International AIDS Conference, Amsterdam.

MCKEGANEY, NEIL, BARNARD, MARINA and BLOOR, MICHAEL (1990) 'A Comparison of HIV-Related Risk Behaviour and Risk Reduction Between Female Street Working Prostitutes and Male Rent Boys in Glasgow', *Sociology of Health and Illness*, 12/3.

MOODIE, T. DUNBAR (1988) 'Migrancy and Male Sexuality on the South African Gold Mines', *Journal of South African Studies*, 14:2, January.

MORBIDITY AND MORTALITY WEEKLY REPORT (1981a) 'Kaposi's Sarcoma and Pneumocystis Pneumonia among Homosexual Men — New York City and California', Atlanta, Centers for Disease Control, 3 July.

MORBIDITY AND MORTALITY WEEKLY REPORT (1981b) 'Follow-Up on Kaposi's Sarcoma and Pneumocystis Pneumonia', Atlanta, Centers for Disease Control, 28 August.

MORBIDITY AND MORTALITY WEEKLY REPORT (1982) 'Update on Kaposi's Sarcoma and Opportunistic Infections in Previously Healthy Persons — United States', Atlanta, Centers for Disease Control, 11 June.

MORBIDITY AND MORTALITY WEEKLY REPORT (1983) 'Immunodeficiency Among Female Partners of Males with Acquired Immune Deficiency Syndrome', Atlanta, Centers for Disease Control, 7 January.

MORBIDITY AND MORTALITY WEEKLY REPORT (1987) 'Antibody to Human Immunodeficiency Virus in Female Prostitutes', Atlanta, Centers for Disease Control, 27 March.

NEJMI, SLIMANE (1986) *Migration and Health*, Geneva, WHO.

NELSON, ALVIN *et al.* (1990) 'Characteristics Associated with a Low Return Rate for HIV Post Test Counseling among Clients in a Community-Based STD Clinic in Los Angeles County', paper presented at International AIDS Conference, San Francisco.

NEWSWEEK (1985a) 'Special Report on AIDS', 12 August.

NEWSWEEK (1985b) 'The AIDS Conflict', 23 September.

NEWSWEEK (1990) 'The Future of Gay America', 12 March.

NORDHEIMER, JON (1987) 'AIDS Specter for Women: The Bisexual Man', New York Times, April, 8.

NORRIS, BARBARA *et al.* (1990) 'Evaluation of Compliance Rate in a Clinic Serving Minority and Low Income Communities [Brooklyn, NY]', paper presented at Sixth International Conference on AIDS, San Francisco.

OLIVEIRA, MARIZA ROEDEL *et al.* (1992) 'Truck Drivers: Evaluation of Attitudes and Knowledge in Relation to HIV/AIDS in Belo Horizonte, Brazil', paper presented at Eighth International Conference on AIDS, Amsterdam.

ONORATO, IDA M. *et al.* (1992) 'High and Rising HIV Incidence in Female Sex Workers in Miami, Florida, Despite Stable HIV Prevalence Rate Over Time', paper presented at Eighth International Conference on AIDS, Amsterdam.

ORUBULOYE, I. O. *et al.* (1992) 'Sexual Behaviour, STDs and HIV/AIDS Transmission: The Role of Long Distance Haulage Drivers and Itinerant Female Hawkers in Nigeria'.

O'SULLIVAN, SUE and PARMAR, PRATIBHA (1992) *Lesbians Talk Safer Sex*, London, Scarlet Press.

PAINTER, THOMAS *et al.* (1992) 'Seasonal Migration and the Spread of AIDS in Mali and Niger', paper presented at Eighth International Conference on AIDS, Amsterdam.

PALTIEL, FREDA L. (1987) 'Women and Mental Health: A Post-Nairobi Perspective', *World Health Statistics Quarterly*, 40/3.

PAPAEVANGELOU, G. *et al.* (1988) 'Education in Preventing HIV Infection in Greek Registered Prostitutes', *Journal of Acquired Immune Deficiency Syndrome*, New York, Raven Press

PATTON, CINDY (1985) 'Heterosexual AIDS Panic: A Queer Paradigm', *Gay Community News*, 9 February.

PATTON, CINDY (1990) *Inventing AIDS*, New York, Routledge.

PATTON, CINDY (1992) 'Containing Safe Sex', in PARKER, ANDREW, SOMER, DORIS, RUSSO, MARY and YAEGER, PATRICIA (Eds) *Nationalisms/Sexualities*, New York and London, Routledge.

PATTON, CINDY and KELLY, JANIS (1987) *Making It: A Woman's Guide to Sex in the Age of AIDS*, Ithaca, Firebrand Press.

PEOPLE MAGAZINE (1988) 'AIDS and the Single Woman', 14 March.

PEOPLE MAGAZINE (1990) 'AIDS: A Woman's Story', 30 July.

PHETERSON, GAIL (1990) 'The Category "Prostitute" in Scientific Inquiry', *Journal of Sex Research*, 27/3. August.

PITT, DAVID (1990) 'Potential Roles for Traditional Health Practitioners and Traditional Birth Attendants in National AIDS Control Programmes', unpublished paper prepared for WHO/GPA consultation in Botswana.

PIVNICK, ANITRA (1991) 'Reproductive Decisions Among HIV-Infected Drug-Using Women: The Importance of Mother-Child Coresidence', *Medical Anthropology Quarterly*.

PIZURKI, HELENA, MEJRA, ALFONSO, BUTTER, IRENE and EWART, LESLIE (1987) *Women as Providers of Health Care*, Geneva, World Health Organization.

PODHISITA, DHAI *et al.* (1992) 'Social/Sexual Networks for HIV Transmission in Thailand', paper presented at Eighth International Conference on AIDS, Amsterdam.

PORTIS, SUKI (1987) 'Needed (For Women and Children)', in CRIMP, D. (Ed.) *AIDS: Cultural Analysis, Cultural Activism*, Cambridge, MA, MIT Press.

RAMPHELE, MAMPHELA (1990) 'Do Women Help Perpetuate Sexism? A Bird's Eye View from South Africa', *Africa Today*, 37/1.

RATNER, MICHAEL (1993) *Crack Pipe as Pimp*, Boston, Lexington Books.

Bibliography

REARDON, JUAN et al. (1992) 'HIV-1 Infection Among Female Injecting Drug Users (IDU) in the San Francisco Bay Area, California', paper presented at Eighth International Conference on AIDS, Amsterdam.

Report on the International Conference on the Implications of AIDS for Mothers and Children (1989) Geneva, World Health Organization.

RICHARDSON, DIANE (1988) *Women and AIDS*, New York, Methuen.

RICHWALD, GARY et al. (1988) 'Are Condom Instructions Readable? Results of a Readability Study', *Public Health Reports*, 103/4, July–August.

RIEDER, INES and RUPPELT, PATRICIA (Eds) (1988) *AIDS: The Women*, Pittsburg, Cleis Press.

RIFKIN, SUSAN B. (1990) *Community Participation in Maternal and Child Health/Family Planning Programmes*, Geneva, World Health Organization.

ROSENBERG, CHARLES E. (1962) *The Cholera Years*, Chicago, University of Chicago Press.

ROYSTON, ERICA and LOPEZ, ALAN D. (1987) 'On the Assessment of Maternal Mortality', *World Health Statistics Quarterly*, 40/3.

RUSSELL, MICHELE A. et al. (1992) 'The Perception of Risk for HIV Infection Among Lesbians in New York City', paper presented at Eighth International Conference on AIDS, Amsterdam.

SAHRAOUI, D. et al. (1992) 'AIDS Prevention Aiming at the North African Population Settled in Workers Centres', paper presented at Eighth International Conference on AIDS, Amsterdam.

SASSE, H. et al. (1992) 'Potential Routes of HIV Transmission Among Women Engaging in Female to Female Sexual Practices', paper presented at Eighth International Conference on AIDS, Amsterdam.

SCHNECK, MARY et al. (1989) 'Reproductive History of HIV Ab+ Women Followed in a Prospective Study in Newark, New Jersey, USA'. paper presented at Fifth International Conference on AIDS, Montreal.

SQUIRE, CORINNE (Ed.) (1993) *Women and AIDS*, London, Sage.

STALL, RON et al (1990) 'Relapse From Safer Sex: The AIDS Behavioral Research Project', paper presented at Sixth International Conference on AIDS, San Francisco.

STANLEY, KENNETH, STJERNSWARD, JAN and KOROLTCHOUK, VALENTIN (1987) 'Women and Cancer', *World Health Statistics Quarterly*, 40/3.

STEVENS, P. CLAY (1988) 'US Women and HIV Infection', *New England Journal of Public Policy*, 4:1, pp. 381–402.

Strategies for Hope see Campbell *and* Williams.

SUNDERLAND, ANN et al. (1989) 'Influence of HIV Infection on Pregnancy Decisions', paper presented at Fifth International Conference on AIDS, Montreal.

TAYLOR, DEANE (1990) 'The Evolution of Dignity: Role of the Cook County Hospital Support Group for HIV Infected Women', paper presented at Sixth International Conference on AIDS, San Francisco.

TIME (1987a) 'In the Grip of the Scourge', 16 February.

TIME (1987b) 'Women and AIDS', 27 April.

TREICHLER, PAULA (1988) 'AIDS, Homophobia, and Biomedical Discourse: An Epidemic of Signification', in CRIMP, DOUGLAS (Ed.) *AIDS: Cultural Analysis/Cultural Activism*, Cambridge, MIT Press.

TRENK, BARBARA SCHERR (1989) 'Hemophilia and AIDS: Where We Stood Before, Where We Stand Now', *AIDS Patient Care*, June.

VAN DUIFHUIZEN, RINSKE et al. (1992) 'AIDS and Mobility: The Impact of International Mobility on the Spread of HIV/AIDS, Need and Possibilities for International Cooperation', paper presented at Eighth International Conference on AIDS, Amsterdam.

VERNON, DIANE (1992) 'A Prevention Program for Tribalized and Urban Bush Negroes', paper presented at Eighth International Conference on AIDS, Amsterdam.

VORAKIPHOKATORN, SAIRUDEE and CASH, R. (1992) 'Factors that Determine Condom Use Among Traditionally High Users: Japanese Men and Commercial Sex Workers (CSW) in Bankok, Thailand', paper presented at Eighth International Conference on AIDS, Amsterdam.

WALDRON, INGRID (1987) 'Patterns and Causes of Excess Female Mortality Among Children', *World Health Statistics Quarterly*, 40/3.

WALLACE, J. I. *et al.* (1992) 'Fellatio Is a Significant Risk Behavior for Acquiring AIDS Among New York City Streetwalking Prostitutes', paper presented at Eighth International Conference on AIDS, Amsterdam.

WARD, HELEN *et al.* (1992) 'Commercial Sex and HIV Risk: A Six Year Study of Female Sex Workers', paper presented at Eighth International Conference on AIDS, Amsterdam.

WENIGER, BRUCE G. *et al.* (1992) 'The HIV Epidemic in Thailand, India, and Neighboring Nations: A Fourth Epidemiologic Pattern Emerges in Asia', paper presented at Eighth International Conference on AIDS, Amsterdam.

WHITESIDE, ALAN (1988) 'Migrant Labor and AIDS in South Africa', paper presented at Global Impact of AIDS Conference, London, 8–10 March.

WILKE, MARTIN and KLEIBER, D. (1992) 'Sexual Behavior of Gay German Sex-Tourists in Thailand', paper presented at Eighth International Conference on AIDS, Amsterdam.

WILLIAMS, GLEN (1990) *From Fear to Hope*, Strategies for Hope Series, No. 1, London, ActionAid.

WIRAWAN, D. N. *et al.* (1992) 'Sexual Behavior and Condom Use of Male Sex Workers and Their Male Tourist Clients in Bali, Indonesia', paper presented at Eighth International Conference on AIDS, Amsterdam.

WIZNIA, ANDREW *et al.* (1989) 'Factors Influencing Maternal Decision-Making Regarding Pregnancy Outcome in HIV Infected Women', paper presented at Fifth International Conference on AIDS, Montreal.

WOMEN'S AIDS NETWORK (1986) 'Lesbians and AIDS: What's the Connection?', San Francisco, San Francisco AIDS Foundation.

WORLD HEALTH ORGANIZATION (1985) *Women, Health and Development: A Report by the Director-General*, Geneva, World Health Organization.

WORLD HEALTH ORGANIZATION (1987) *Evaluation of the Strategy for Health for All by the Year 2000*, Volumes 1–7, Geneva, World Health Organization.

WORLD HEALTH ORGANIZATION (1988) *From Alma-Ata to the Year 2000: Reflections at the Midpoint*, Geneva, World Health Organization.

WORLD HEALTH ORGANIZATION (1989a) *Broadcasters' Questions and Answers on AIDS*, Geneva, World Health Organization.

WORLD HEALTH ORGANIZATION (1989b) *The Reproductive Health of Adolescents*, Geneva, World Health Organization.

WORLD HEALTH ORGANIZATION (1990) *The Work of WHO, 1988–1989: The Biennial Report of the Director-General*, Geneva, World Health Organization.

Index

Note: 'n.' after a page reference denotes the number of a note on that page.

158